Flanagan Speaks!

Dialogues on

Pyramid Power, Health & Healing & Spiritual Awakening

With

Dr. Patrick Flanagan
&
Deepak Chopra
Patrick Timpone
Paula Peterson
& Joseph Marcello

Compiled & Edited

By
Joseph Andrew Marcello

ISBN: 9781070450858

Printed in the United States of America

TABLE OF CONTENTS

DIALOGUE WITH DEEPAK CHOPRA

Deepak Chopra: Don't be offended by what I'm going to say. . .so Patrick represents the architect (archetype) of the Fool, he represents the architect (archetype) of the Child; he represents the architect (archetype) of a Wizard, he represents the architect (archetype) of a Sage—and he represents the architect (archetype) of a Trickster (laughter). So, that's a lot of things, right?— all rolled into one.

Patrick Flanagan: Wow—you sure nailed me. It's interesting, because of Jean Houston's book about The Wizard. ..my wife, Stephanie, and I had a huge Theme Camp called Emerald City, and I was the Wizard of Oz, and we had the biggest lasers on earth out there. It was the first huge, giant Theme Camp. Going backward, I was born in the Wizard wave spellof the Mayan calendar, a yellow, electric warrior in the Wizard Wave Spell—I just thought that was an interesting coincidence.

I was a premature baby, and I just couldn't wait to get out, you know, and get moving in the world; I remember laying in my crib and wiggling my toes, and I remember very distinctly thinking, "I hate growing up baby bodies; I hate it—because it's going to take me so long before I could get back to work again. It was very, very clear.

DC: Fast forward to when you're 17, and you have already become a consultant to the NSA, CIA, NASA,

Tufts University, the Office of Naval Research and the Aberdeen Proving Grounds in the Deparmtent of Unconvential Weapons and Warfare, and you develop all these amazing technologies for the CIA at the age of 17.

PF: Yes. When Admiral Red Braeburn was director of the CIA, I won this award, which was the Gold Plate Award—it was an achievement award. The Gold Plate people are in Washington D.C.; I don't know a lot about them, but we went to San Diego when I was 17 and I received this award—it was just a gold plate—but it was a nice gold plate. . .And sitting next to me on this side was Edward Teller—

DC: I know who Edward Teller was—

PD: He got the award for inventing the atomic bomb. Admiral Red Braeburn got the award because he invented the Polaris submarine, and then Secretary of State Pete Peters was over here getting the award, and the guy who discovered the sculpture of viruses, Maury Gellman, got the award. We were all sitting there together getting the same award. Red Braeburn and Pete Peterson said "Son, we want to send you to any university you want in the world – don't worry about getting in, we'll get you in." This was 1962— they said, "We'll give you $165,000 a year for an allowance, to spend as you want, and we'll pay for all your other expenses.

DC: What had you invented that got you to this point?

PF: I had invented a Neurophone—well, the only

problem was that I could read 15,000 words a minute, and I didn't like sleep because I couldn't learn when I was asleep. I had read this science fiction book written by Hugo Gernsback, head of Gernsback Publications, a worldwide scientific publishing company. He wrote a 1911 science fiction book, and he had this device he could put on his head and transfer knowledge into his head while he slept. I thought—wow, I can learn while I'm sleeping if I had (something like) that. Hugo Gernsback predicted all sorts of universals—radar, television, all kinds of things; six months after I read that book I invented the Neurophone, which is a device that programs knowledge into the long-term memory (system) of the brain while you sleep. (Inaudible. . .) Hugo Gernsback, at the age of 90-something, wrote me a letter thanking me for inventing the last item that he had predicted in his book that had yet to be invented.

DC: (inaudible question about patents)

PF: I don't like getting patents, because patents reveal all your secrets—your knowledge. . .I have a few patents, but I have over 300 inventions. The government put my Neurophone under secrecy—they thought it had a weapons use—and Red Braeburn said to me, "Son, if you ever get in trouble with the government, you just call the CIA and you leave a message for me and I'll call you back within 24 hours, and I'll take care of whatever the government does to you." And so I said, "Okay, thanks a lot," and he said, "If I do that, then you'll owe me a favor—and you have to do whatever I tell you to do," That's pretty heavy.

They had my Neurophone under secrecy, so I called up the CIA one night and the guy says, (voice becoming Clint Eastwood-like), "May I help you?"—and I said, (equally Eastwood-like),"I want to leave a message for Red Braeburn." By that time he was head of NSA—the National Security Administration. And the voice on the other end of the phone said, "Never heard of him." I said that he was the director of the CIA, and he said, "Still never heard of him." And I said, "Well, he said if I left a message here he'd call me back"—and the guy said, "You can leave a message here for anyone you want, but I won't guarantee you that they'll ever call you back." So anyway, Red Braeburn called me back, and he got my Neurophone out of secrecy—and he asked me to do *him* a favor. The favor I did him was to invent an electronic encryption device for voice communications that could never be undone—in other words no one would ever be able to de-code it. We had a few little things going back and forth that I can't talk about.

DC: One of the most remarkable inventions you had was to communicate with underwater life. . .

PF: Yeah. . .dolphins. During the Vietnam war I worked for a Naval Ordnance Test Station out of China Lake, California; it was called NOTS—they say that NOTS makes Area 51 look like a children's playground. We had dolphins in Hawaii—and this is before you had computer chips or integrated circuits, so we built a computer that translated human speech into dolphin language-whistles, and then translated dolphin whistles back into human speech. We were

4

developing a common language between man and dolphin. Also, we used my Neurophone on the dolphins. The ideal was to develop a 500-word vocabulary—in any language, there are 500 word which will enable you to communicate with anyone in that language and to expand your knowledge and vocabulary. The idea was that we were going to teach the dolphins 500 words and we would talk to each other. We got up to 35 words. B.F. Skinner, the animal behaviorist, said that all animals are just stimulus-response organisms, including humans; but he said that animals can't think. We would tell the dolphins, swim out, go through a hoop, touch a ball, go get a ring and bring it back, and the dolphin would do that. And the dolphin would tell the human divers to do the same thing, and they would. It was like a game. But Skinner said, if you tell the dolphin to swim through the hoop and touch the ball, and then, halfway there, say—no, touch the ball first and then swim through the hoop, that will confuse the dolphin, and he won't be able to do anything. But) we proved him wrong. The dolphins were *way* ahead of us—they were *so* smart.

DC: So the US Navy (inaudible)

PF: Yes—my partner, Dr. Wiley Matthew, who was a Tufts University professor

JOSEPH MARCELLO

THE HUNZA SECRETS OF
THE FOUNTAIN OF YOUTH

A Conversation with Dr. G. Patrick Flanagan

by Paula Peterson

Patrick Flanagan, PhD, avid inventor and author of the bestselling books *Pyramid Power* and *Toward a New Alchemy*, is a leader in the fascinating field of structured water.

Flanagan was a child prodigy whose debut upon the public scene began at age twelve when he submitted his latest project to a science fair. It was a device to detect atomic bombs and guided missiles. The government took control of his invention, but Flanagan's precocious genius was established. The rest, as they say, is history. In 1997, he was voted Scientist of the Year by the International Association for New Science.

Besides his groundbreaking work on identifying and duplicating the benefits of "youthing" waters, Flanagan's work spans inventions like the Neurophone — a helmet-like device that enables deaf people to hear — and technology that was used during the Viet Nam war for training dolphins to recognize and report the country of origin of approaching submarines. In fact, much of the work Flanagan has done, including the dolphin communication research, has been co-opted by the government and is no longer available even to him

The author interviewed Dr. Flanagan in person at his

home.

Paula: When did you begin to take an interest in water?

Patrick: It began when I was still in my teens. I met Dr. Coanda of Stanford University, an amazing man — you can read about him in the Encyclopedia Britannica — who built the first jet airplane in 1911. He also is known as the father of fluid dynamics. During his lifetime, he obtained five hundred patents on fluid amplifiers.

Dr. Coanda was in remarkable health when I met him — he lived to be one-hundred and one. I myself was already a student of health and nutrition and was a pure vegan at the time.

He told me that based upon what he had learned about me, he had decided to share his research with me so that I could continue it. This was because he believed he could not finish it himself in his own lifetime.

He went on to say that the legend of the Fountain of Youth was true, and that there was scientific fact to back it up.

There are five places on Earth, he told me, where people were in extremely good health and lived to be over 100 years old: Hunza Land (in the Karkorum Mountains north of Pakistan), a place in Ecuador, another place in Peru, the county of Georgia in Russia, and a place in Mongolia.

In these locations, the people all have very different diets. The one thing they have in common is the water.

Paula: Most of us don't learn in school that there can be differences in water.

Patrick: Yes, in school we learn that water is the same everywhere in the world: It freezes at zero degrees [centigrade], boils at 100 degrees, and has a certain viscosity and surface tension.

But those are only the average qualities of water. Dr. Coanda said water was different everywhere in the world and that he could predict, just from analyzing the water they drank, the average lifespan of the people who lived in any given area.

Coanda had gone to Hunza Land at the turn of the century. To get there, he had to hike for three months through jungles, climb mountain peaks, and cross rope bridges. While he was there, he found that the Hunza's water came from glaciers that were millions of years old.

There were certain characteristics of Hunza water that Coanda tried his whole life to duplicate. But he never succeeded. He told me, "You, Patrick, will invent a machine that will create this kind of water anywhere in the world. You will save many, many lives." He then gave me the characteristics of Hunza water.

Paula: Do the significant characteristics go beyond the mineral content?

Patrick: Well, he had no idea which characteristics were

significant. He thought that it could even have been the cold temperatures, or the altitude — Hunza Land is a valley at 8000 feet elevation, surrounded by some of the tallest mountains in the world. These mountains have ice-blue glaciers, and this is where their water comes from.

The Hunza people themselves claimed that their secret of health and longevity came from drinking the glacier waters that were filled with all these minerals from the glacial silt. There actually was a well in the area that had clear water, but none of the residents would drink from it — they saved that water for the tourists.

.So at age seventeen—in parallel with everything else that was going on at the time—I started my own research into water. I tried everything: magnetic treatments, alternating different frequency fields, electrolysis—about anything that you could imagine in order to create anomalous properties in water.

I discovered that when I put rubies, quartz crystals, and other gemstones in water and let it sit, that changed the structure of the water and lowered the surface tension. Each night, I would put a brandy snifter next to my bed filled with distilled water containing the crystals. In the morning, I would drink this water, being careful not to cause any turbulence —because even though crystals change water dramatically, all the structuring goes away if you shake it, stir it, or bump it.

Paula: It's that fragile?

Patrick: Yes. Magnets are the same way. I found that crystals have a very orderly matrix of electrical charges, both positive and negative. They will align themselves to the crystal structure of precious stones and then extend out into the water.

Then I reasoned that if I could make the crystals small enough that I put into the water, the change in structure would lower the surface tension and be maintained even through drinking or shaking.

Paula: Before we go on with this explanation, could you please tell us what is meant by the surface tension of water?

Patrick: Surface tension has to do with penetration. For example, if you put a drop of water on a piece of paraffin and look at it from the side, that drop of water will form a nearly perfect sphere because it cannot penetrate the paraffin. But if you put a drop of water on a quartz crystal, it penetrates 100 percent and the drop goes flat.

The surface tension of water is also called the "webbing angle of water." It is well known in food science that every food and substance has a certain webbing angle of water. If the substance is above a certain angle, it cannot wet the food. As an example, it's difficult to mash potatoes with cold water, as they will only clump up. Boiling the water causes the surface tension to go way down, which makes it much easier to mash the potatoes.

Ordinary water has a high surface tension of about 73 dynes per centimeter — a dyne is a unit of force. Boiling water can get as low as 37 dynes. Hunza water has a surface tension of about 67 dynes — and also a different viscosity and a slightly different freezing and boiling point.

Paula: How does all this work in our body?

Patrick: The cells in our body have to be fully wetted with water in order to exchange compounds, getting rid of toxins generated by their own metabolism, and absorbing nutrients. If the cells are not wetted, nutrients and toxins cannot penetrate the surface of the cell. And since the cells are covered with protein lipid membranes— which are fatty acids, and as we know, oil and water do not mix — it's important that the surface tension of the water around our cells water be low enough to allow penetration.

So the Hunza water has a low surface tension. Furthermore, the minerals in the Hunza water are in colloidal suspension. The really cloudy minerals drop out — those are not colloids, and are suspended only while the water is in motion.

Paula: So you are saying that a colloidal mineral is different than other minerals?

Patrick: Yes. Basically, colloidal minerals are more bio-available. In fact, they are what the body needs and uses. The body has to work really hard to separate minerals out of compounds. For example, if you take magnesium chloride in order to get magnesium, your body has to separate the magnesium out of the chloride before it can use it.

But a colloidal mineral is suspended in the solution (not dissolved).[3] When the suspension medium is water, the minerals must be small enough, and must carry a strong enough electrical charge, so that they don't coagulate and repel each other.

Colloidal minerals also have a negative electrical charge, which is very important. The higher the negative charge, the more of the mineral will suspend in water without dropping out. So colloidal minerals have to be tiny and have a strong negative charge.

Consequently, I realized that the secret of Hunza water was in the tiny size of the colloidal minerals. And I found that these minerals were mostly silica. Silica is an essential mineral for the human body. It helps to produce collagen: the matrix that holds our skin together.

Paula: Is that the same kind of silica that's found in quartz crystal?

Patrick: Yes. Quartz crystal is silica in a crystal form. There is also amorphous silica, which is totally non-crystalline.

By the time I had worked for almost 30 years on this, trying to figure out how to make Hunza water, I had become famous for the book *Pyramid Power*, and was a featured speaker all over the world, with television specials and a movie made about me called *Outer Space Connections*.

In due course, my wife and I went through a hermit stage and I withdrew from the public eye. We moved to Sedona, Arizona, and bought a house on forty acres of land. The house was fifteen miles up a dirt road that had no name. Trees completely surrounded our property.

We essentially isolated ourselves for fourteen years, and it was during these years in isolation, along with practicing specific spiritual disciplines, that I made some of my most revolutionary discoveries.

Paula: Which discoveries were your most important?

Patrick: I created Crystal Energy, which was my first concentrated colloidal solution. When added to water, Crystal Energy restructures it.

We went on a six-month fast on water and juices supplemented with Crystal Energy. At the end of the six-month fast, I had lost 45 pounds and my wife lost about 25 pounds. Friends who visited us were astounded and amazed that we looked like teenagers, even though I was 45 years old at this time. I'm 58 now.

Paula: I have to say that you look extraordinarily healthy!

Patrick: Thank you. I know it's from using Crystal

Energy and also from the water I later developed, called silica-hydride, using microclusters of silica

We had the Microcluster® water tested at different universities. These tests showed that our product was little spheres. Not only that, the little spheres would group together and form bigger spheres in which other things could be inserted.

For example, flax seed oil goes rancid faster than any other known oil because it is highly polyunsaturated and can easily be attacked by oxygen. We found that when we mixed flax seed oil with the microcluster powder it would not go rancid, not even after two years of sitting on the shelf!

Paula: That's amazing. What was your next stage of discovery?

Patrick: I found a way to make silica Buckyballs in my lab through using nanotechnology. Buckyballs, named after Buckminster Fuller, are formations of structured carbon made up of tiny little spheres that look like soccer balls. Further findings proved that atomic nuclei could be trapped inside the Buckyballs and used as a carrier for transporting pharmaceuticals into the cells.

The minerals in Hunza water were like Buckyballs, only they were made of silica instead of carbon. When they were added to water, they lowered the surface tension. My technology reduces the surface tension of water to 28 dynes per centimeter. Pure ethyl alcohol is 27 dynes per centimeter. This means that this restructured water has the solvent capabilities of ethyl alcohol. It's really quite remarkable.

In subsequent research, we took hundreds of people off the streets to do darkfield microscope studies of their blood. We found that most people's blood looked like sewers: The cells were all clumped together with free-radical damage, and sometimes we'd see little parasites swimming around.

After taking the silica-hydride product, their blood cells would become beautiful and discrete again, the parasites would disappear, and all the damage from free radicals would be gone — all within fifteen minutes of taking only two capsules.

Most people are walking around in a chronic state of dehydration where their blood is clumped together. It's a condition in modern people that eventually leads to plaque on arteries, heart attacks, and nutritional deficiencies caused from a build-up of toxins that the body cannot eliminate.

Paula: Now, that's something that intrigues me. I learned that most people are dehydrated most of the time, but that after a certain period of dehydration they don't seem to crave water. Why is that?

Patrick: No one knows why our sense of thirst seems to disappear as we get older. When we're babies, we know immediately when we need water, and we cry for it. And yet as we get older we can become severely dehydrated and not even know it.

To make matters worse, the surface tension of the bodily fluids goes up as we age, and again, no one knows why. Dehydration is one of the major indicators of the aging process. On top of that, in today's world, various factors like electro-magnetic pollution, unhealthy diets, and, in particular, poor water destroy the electrical charge of blood cells.

Studies show that silica-hydride is the greatest hydrating agent ever discovered. In our studies we gave people silica hydride, and in four weeks the average person on the study reversed age — as far as hydration is concerned — by five years.

Paula: Is there evidence that this kind of water was more available on the Earth at one time?

Patrick: Yes, and there are many theories about that. A friend of mine who is a biblical scholar says that in the Bible it tells of a time when people lived to be hundreds of years old, and that there was a constant light everywhere — everything was lit up.

Some scientists believe that the Earth was once surrounded by ice crystals high up in the stratosphere. The ice crystals refracted sunlight and blocked cosmic rays that are damaging to our DNA. Cosmic rays are passing through us all the time, now.

Paula: Does that have anything to do with "the firmament" that is mentioned in the Book of Genesis? It has been hypothesized that the firmament was an atmosphere made of water.

Patrick: Yes. That's what it was. The theory is that the Great Flood of Noah's time — which is recorded in many ancient texts throughout the world — was caused by the ice crystals coagulating, as colloids tend to do. And so it rained for forty days and forty nights, which flooded the entire Earth. Even prior to the flood, rain occasionally may have come from the firmament, making healthy water much more available in those days.

Paula: I am aware of theories humans once ate only flowers, leaves, and fruits, and that something of a catastrophic nature happened that destroyed nearly all living things. According to these theories, surviving humans became nomadic, since much of the Earth was then uninhabitable and there was less available food, and humans began to eat the animals.

Patrick: Yes. There are theories that humans did not eat meat prior to the Great Flood, which is another possible answer to why humans had longer life spans. In certain areas above and below the equator, where our ancestors originally came from, humans lived in jungles where they simply reached out and picked their food. Since their food was so abundant, they didn't have to work for it, and so for the most part they played.

When Earth's climate began to change, and the rainforests started drying up, fruit became less available. So humans began scavenging for food outside the forests. Not only that, the earth's axis was once straight up and down, which caused spring to pervade all year long all over the planet.

Paula: You certainly have lived a fascinating life. Can you share with us any new research on water that's particularly exciting for you right now?

Patrick: Yes. I recently discovered another component in Hunza water that I didn't know about. I found that Hunza water had hydride ions, which are hydrogen atoms with a negative charge plus an extra electron. A hydrogen atom normally has only one proton and one electron, but it can actually take on and carry an extra electron. That extra electron is of the right potential to neutralize free radicals and participate in all the thousands and thousands of chemical reactions in the body that require extra electrons.

By using a laser and other techniques, I discovered that these hydride ions — or H-minus ions — are in Hunza water, and also in the juices of all fresh raw, living fruits and vegetables.

Paula: I'm so glad you said that. Being a health educator for several years, I have encouraged others to eat raw, living foods.

Patrick: We should all eat raw food, period, and no cooked food. When food is processed, dried, or cooked, the first thing that leaves the food are these important hydride ions.

Paula: The enzymes are destroyed, too.

Patrick: Well, the enzymes can't function without the H-minus ions, and that's why the enzymes stop functioning and die from heating. I think it's the most important nutrient. However, it's also the one that disappears the fastest. Most people are very deficient in it. I've known many people who were dying of cancer who went on a raw food, raw juice only diet and cured themselves, because they were giving their body all the right nutrients. These extra electrons are the most abundant in freshly made, raw juices.

When I discovered hydride ions and figured out a way to impregnate water with them, I started drinking the water. It gave me so much energy and made me feel so good that I eventually developed a very stable form of microclustered water with H-minus ions.

Those who took the water reported miracles--unbelievable things. One woman reported restoration of her nerve-damaged arm after she'd had no feeling in it for fifteen years. Diabetics have reported the return of feelings in their legs after having lost it for twenty years.

The remarkable thing about all of this is that it has been such a win/win situation. It has done great things for so many people.

Paula: Thank you, Patrick, for being so generous with your time today. Your discoveries are truly remarkable and continue to offer hope to so many.

PYRAMIDS, PENTAGONS &
THE PATH OF AWAKENING

A Dialogue with Patrick Flanagan

by

Joseph Marcello

JM: Let's go back, Patrick, to the days just prior to your meeting Nick Edwards, and just what you were spending your time doing.

PF: I had written my book, *Pyramid Power.* and I decided to get it published, and I couldn't find anyone who was willing to publish the book; publishers said they didn't think it would sell, and so I borrowed $5000 and I published it the first time, 5000 copies of *Pyramid Power* in hardback; they cost me a dollar each and I sold them for, I think, back then—$10. And it took off like wildfire—it was extremely successful, and over the next few years I sold a million and a half copies of *Pyramid Power*.

JM: Are we right in saying that this was the first contemporary book on the subject?

PF: Oh, absolutely, the first contemporary book on the subject. Although it had been mentioned in a book by Ostrander, in which she addressed pyramids and spoke about a man in Czechoslovakia who had patented a pyramid razor blade sharpener. I had been doing research on orgone energy; I had built orgone energy accumulators, and had experienced and measured all kinds of energy changes from those. And when I read the Ostrander book, I started building pyramids out of cardboard and pyramid orgone energy accumulators and pyramids. I found that combining the two was absolutely a compatible synthesis.

JM: And that would have been Sheila Ostrander and Lynne Schroeder's *Psychic Discoveries Behind the Iron Curtain* correct?

PF: Exactly.

JM: And that's when you were first awakened to the possibilities of pyramid energy – and you tried to combine this with Wilhelm Reich's orgone?

PF: I did, yes.

JM: And did you find that a compatible synthesis?

PF: I did, absolutely.

JM: Because I had read—perhaps erroneously—I have a couple of books on how to create your own orgone accumulators as well, but haven't explored it—that it's actually possible to overaccumulate and to create a negative effect on the human system.

PF: I disagree with that—yes, there is something called 'DOR' which is negative orgone energy. Orgone accumulators do not accumulate DOR.

JM: So this sounds like an inspiration which has yet to be promulgated publicly—at least this is the first I've ever heard of it—combining these two protocols.

PF: It's true.

JM: Is there a reason you haven't purveyed that?

PF: No, that should at some point be revealed in my new books on these energies.

JM: So then you began to experiment—you were a scientist of some kind, and you could actually construct accurate models.

PF: Yes.

JM: And what did you make them from?

PF: I made them from cardboard.

JM: And you experienced an effect right off?

PF: Yes, but not only that, but as a scientist I had developed techniques of measuring the energies of the orgone box and then the pyramids. My technique for measuring this was a differential thermometer; my tests had demonstrated—which is what Albert Einstein had pervasively demonstrated—was that the temperature in the orgone accumulator was always a couple of degrees Centigrade higher than the temperature than in the environment outside the accumulator—and this theoretically is impossible.

And so I built what is called a wheatstone bridge, using thermal diodes; I built a bridge so that I could neutralize the two diodes in the room temperature so that they were equal, and I put one diode inside the pyramid and one outside, and invariably the diode inside the pyramid and or the orgone accumulator would show a positive temperature differential – that it would always be higher inside the accumulator or the pyramid than it would outside.

That was my method of measurement, and it was extremely accurate – much more accurate the method of measurement that Wilhelm Reich undertook.

JM: It must have been something of an astonishment —a 'Eureka!' moment to find such a concrete read-out of the pyramid or orgone energy.

PF: It *was* a 'Eureka!' moment, and remember, from the age of 8 forward I was a child prodigy and I worked for the government; the government took one of my inventions when I was 12 years old, and so I'm unique in that I'm making discoveries as a child that have never been seen before on this planet.

JM: Anything that we might be familiar with today?

PF: Well, the first thing, when I was 12 years old, was that I invented an atomic-bomb missile-detector and won a science fair with it; the Houston All-Grade science fair, which went all the way through college. The following Monday I was in study hall in the 7th grade and the principal came over the loud speaker and said, "Will Patrick Flanagan come to my office immediately – the Pentagon is on the telephone."

And I went to the office and there was a 5-star general on the line, and he wanted to know how I knew about all the nuclear testing and intercontinental ballistic missiles that they had fired and where they had fired them from. And I told him about my science fair project and they sent a team of 15 people from Mike Patterson Air Force Base to Houston and took my invention away, and made my father sign one of those agreements that said if I revealed anything to anyone other than the government about my invention that I could be tried for treason, and that if convicted that the penalty was death.

So that was the beginning, and that science fair project of course hit all the papers—I still have copy of me with my science fair project.

You can't explain where this all came from – when I was 8 years old I was designing and building vacuum tube radio receivers and transmitters; I got my general class amateur radio license, I was sending Morse code at 33 words per minute, and I was designing and building all my own equipment and antennas and such. And then when I was 13 years old I designed and built the Neurophone, which is a device that transmits information directly into long term memory in the brain, and which balances the left and right hemispheres of the brain creating brain-phase coherence between the two hemispheres and increases IQ—I invented that just coming on to my 13th birthday. Now, these are inventions that no one else in the world has ever seen before—the missile detector and the Neurophone—so I wrote my own patent, I went and studied at the library, and the patent office refused to give a patent because they said there was no trial or art. Of course, I said, "Isn't that what an invention is – something that no one has ever seen before. but of course, 99.9999 percent of the inventions for which people apply for patents are improvements on pre-existing ideas—things that are already known.

It took 40 years before a scientist at the University of Virginia discovered that there is an organ inside the head that responds to a Neurophone ultrasonic energy and that that organ is an organ of balance but it also turns out that it is a vestigial organ of hearing for all ultrasonic sound, and that it is the hearing organ of whales and dolphins. Ultimately, when the patent office and closed the file, by the time I was 19 I was able to afford an attorney and the patent office said if I came to the patent office with my invention and I was able to make a deaf employee who worked at the patent office hear—that the patent office would re-open the file—which has never been done in the history of that office. They would give me my original filing date as well as my patent.

So, when I was 19 I flew to the patent office with my invention and my lawyer, and we went in—and we put the Neurophone on the head of this employee, who had been stone deaf for 15 years; he happened to love opera music, and back then they only had 78 r.p.m. record players, and we put a 78 r.p.m. Of Maria Callas singing on and he heard for the first time, and he broke down in tears sobbing, and everyone in the patent office started crying; and they re-opened my file, issued me my original patent filing date and gave me my patent. Later on the patent office gave me an award for that, because it has never happened before or since that they have done such a thing.

These devices are still available today—we manufacture and sell them. The government and national security reviews all patent applications, and if they think your invention has possible military uses they take the invention. So the military then started doing things to prevent me from manufacturing and selling the device.

I applied for a second patent on the device and they put it under "secrecy" just like the guided missile detector. When I was 17 years old I received an offer to come to San Diego to receive something called the Gold Plate Award of the American Academy of Achievement; for my invention and achievement. So I went to San Diego with my parents, and sitting at the table with me, receiving the same award that I was receiving, for their achievements, were Dr. Edward Teller, who invented the hydrogen bomb, Admiral Red Raeburn, who was director in charge of the CIA, for inventing the polar submarine, Maury Gellman, Nobel Prize-winner for his discoveries of the genetics of viruses.

Admiral Raeburn said to me, "Son, we would like to put you in any university in the world you want— don't worry about getting in—we'll put you there; we'll give you a $175,000 a year allowance in addition to paying for your schooling—and that was in 1962;

and he said, "You can go to school as long as you want, get as many degrees as you want, and when you're done, we want you to work for the CIA for 5 years, at which time we will release you and you can do what you want to do.

And so I talked around to various friends, and they said "They will never let go of you – ever, if you do that." At that time I was making more money than my father because I was working for the Pentagon think tank, and consulting. So I turned down the offer from Raeburn and the CIA; and so Raeburn said, "I'll tell you what, son—let's go into what we call the 'Favors' program"; and I said, "What is that?" And he said, "If you have any troubles with the government, I'll do you a favor, and no matter what the problem is, I'll fix it." And then he said, "And then you'll have to a favor for me—whatever that favor is, you have to do it," and I said, "Okay, that sounds fine with me."

In the meantime, my second patent application on the Neurophone had been put under secrecy by the government, and so Red Raeburn said, "Call the CIA, leave a message for me, and I'll call you back within 24 hours." And so I'm getting frustrated by this, so I called the CIA one night and I said, "I want to leave a message for Admiral Red Raeburn," and the guy said, "Never heard of him,"—by then he had gone on to become the director of the National Security Agency, so I said, "He was director of your agency," and the guy said "Still never heard of him." And I said, "Well, he told me I could leave a message for him and he'd call me back within 24 hours," and the guy said, "You can leave a message for anyone you want with me, but I can't guarantee that they'll call you back." I said, "That's fair enough, so I left a message for Rae Braeburn, and sure enough, he called me back, and I said, "This patent application is under secrecy, and I want to get it out of secrecy." He said, "Done." And I said, "Okay."

So they took it out of secrecy and issued my patent. What he didn't tell me was that—just because they took it out of secrecy—didn't mean that they would allow me to manufacture and sell it. But that said, he then went on to ask me for a little favor, and that 'Favors' program went on for years.

I was doing and inventing things that no Ph.D. In the world ever dreamed of, when I was a kid. I was beyond that. When I wrote and published 'Pyramid Power' they were stalking me, preventing me from manufacturing the Neurophone, blocking me at every stage – and I can prove that—I got a call from a guy in the CIA, and he said, "Son, the best thing you ever did for yourself is write and publish 'Pyramid Power', and I said, "Why is that?", and he said, "They think you went off the deep end, and they let go their reins on you because they don't consider you to be a threat anymore."

JM: So they didn't consider that scientifically viable,

PF: Exactly. . .

JM: And therefore they considered you a quack.

PF: And so, my whole life changed – and at that point I was able to put the Neurophone on the market and we've been selling it ever since. The thing about the Neurophone being a hearing aid is that the original model I had was so extremely powerful that it put 3,000 volts across these electrodes that you put on your head, and the electrodes were insulated by mylar tape so that they didn't shock you, but it produced very, very powerful ultrasonic sound. And it turns out this fellow at the University of Virginia duplicated the Neurophone in 1997 and showed that that profoundly deaf people *can* hear with it, but the power level has to be extremely high, and the Neurophones we have on the market don't have that much power; but that said, they still cause all this phenomena, like full brain-phase coherence, it increases IQ, it transmits sound information directly into long term memory in the brain, it increases the neural networks in the temporal lobes of the brain.

The Neurophone creates a kind of bridge for the deaf to access the world of frequency, and it stimulates

there is a connection between the pituitary and the pineal gland which is shown in Tibetan anatomy which is depicted as a musical instrument, with a little, tiny channel between the two glands—a lyre—and what happens is that when the spinal builds up a certain pressure and the spinal fluid starts oscillating back and forth between the pineal and pituitary, it creates a powerful musical sound in the head—it creates a note—it's a very, very loud tone, and sometimes when it goes off, it cuts off the field of your own hearing, and that's when the two glands are really communicating and opening up your third eye.

JM: Well this sounds very intimate to an experience I've had all my life, especially after kriya yoga practice made me aware of it—there was a constant internal vibratory sound that was always audible to me –

PF: Yes, I have it all the time –

JM: – and I think that it's audible to everybody, but that everybody is addicted to thought, and they obscure it by constant thinking or 'self-talk'; and when I'm quiet—which is easy for me to do now—there it is, always there.

PF: Yeoh.

JM: And if it is focused upon—I believe it is one and the same with the traditional practices known as the Shabd or the Word; and you're right, if it is focused upon, it does become magnified—even to the point where it will obliterate ancillary sounds – and even lift you out of your body, if you go that far.

PF: Yes. My wife has just recently become aware of that sound—and it can be disturbing unless you know what that sound is.

(Patrick's wife, Stephanie, enters the discussion)

SF: I'm sorry to interject, but I've been hearing your conversation and I've been so wanting to understand what this ongoing ambient sound in my head that never goes away is.

JM: Are you wanting me to address it from my own experience

SF: Do you mind, Patrick

PF: No – please!

JM: Hi Stephanie. . .

SF: Hi Joseph. . .

JM: It can be a little unsettling, if you have the feeling that it can get out of hand –

SF: --right—

JM: – and de-stabilize your cognitive balance?

SF: Exactly. . .

JM: And what I've discovered, which I think will console you, is that eventually, once you've been able to wrap yourself around it and experiment a bit— provided it's not merely a case of inflammation in your Eustachian tubes or your brain somewhere. . .

SF: Yes. . .

JM: And I think you would have other symptoms that would manifest if it was inflammation, or pre-fever or infection of some kind. To share an example—when I was a kid at summer camp, I happened to have very strongly slapped at a mosquito that was on the side of my head, and I actually ruptured my ear drum by the transmitted air vibration from my palm.

SF: – wow. . .

JM: – and for several days thereafter—because I was an avid swimmer and I would swim every day in the lake—I could hear this rather intrusive high pitch from one side of my nervous system, which turned out to be caused by the sound-distortion produced by the passage of air through the very fine rupture in my eardrum. And that healed and I didn't lose any hearing; but I'm mentioning that as an example of a persistent sonic intrusion with an organic basis, that isn't the same phenomenon as the audible flow of one's life energy which I'm speaking about. So I can't say what you may be experiencing. . .

SF: I know it's not anything like that – no. . .no

JM: This is what I have never read even in some of the most advanced Kriya books and esoteric meditation texts—there's a whole tradition in the east of meditation on the 'sacred sound" called the Shabd, and it's considered higher than any other meditative form because it's considered a direct emanation of the Godhead or the Source Energy of the universe, without any intermediary, which, while there are many eastern texts, why, in the west, they describe it in the Bible in John 1:1 as the Word: in the beginning— at the start of all things—was the Word, which is another way of saying the sound –

SF: Yes, I'm very aware of that. . .

JM: —or the vibration of the creative force. And that had to happen because—let's say with me, as a composer – if I don't strike a note on the piano or the guitar, I'm going to be sitting in silence, right? I may be feeling all sorts of things—urges and feelings—but unless I create a differential—that is, unless I cause something within that silence to start vibrating—I'm not going to have any music. So, the Godhead, wanting to express its own richness, struck that initial – and continuing—vibratory impetus into effect, and that's called the Word. Is that something which you can understand?

SF: Oh yes, I'm very much into "In the beginning was the Word and the Word was with God. . ." – yes.

JM: And we can't draw breath without that word. I mean that the Word is the life-energy itself as it vibrates through space and vibrates through the human nervous system. It's your life-fuel; you're still with me?

SF: Absolutely.

JM: Okay—so it's very easy to hear that, as I telling Patrick, provided you know how to be still; but that's a big provision—and most people I meet don't know how to be still—and by 'being still' I mean to stop talking to themselves within their own minds.

SF: Right –

JM: And, actually, to have no thought—

SF: Right—

JM: A state of no thinking. At that point, awakening

begins to happen; at least it does within me—not only awakening to what's going on in one's environment, but also awakening to what's going on within your own being.

SF: Right –

JM: So you're not talking, either aloud or internally, anymore—and projecting thoughts or dialogues; you're really the Divine Listener at this point.

SF: Yes, very much so, very much so. . .

JM: And you really begin to hear what you did not hear before—you hear the sounds underneath the sounds when you go out into Nature, you hear the trickling of the stream far away, beneath the bird calls; you hear all sorts of things because you're finally quiet for a change.

SF: Oh, I just crave quiet—like at night—I just so love being in bed, in pitch dark, with nothing around me and going into this space—it's like my favorite thing to do.

JM: Well, I can identify or empathize with you, because, at least where I am now spiritually, I consider the whole evolution of the self and personality—your "Stephanie"—and my "Joseph", and Patrick's "Patrick"—the development of those selves –

SF: Yes—

JM: —is a very stressful phenomenon –

Sf: —yes, yes, yes—

JM: —because they are really intrusions upon the ultimate reality –

SF: —yes, that's right I totally, totally have been receiving this –

JM: But they're not to be abused, or killed off, the way the easterners suppose, because that only winds up by committing spiritual suicide. There's a reason that they exist—so that I can talk to you and you can wrap your arms around Patrick and through them we're able to relate to each other—right?

SF: Mm hm, mm hm. . .

JM: But they have usurped their rightful place, and they have tried to cover the entire field of consciousness.

SF: Right, right. . .

JM: And that is a stress—even though we may not be aware of that stress: most people on earth right now think that the ego is all of it.

SF: Right. . .

JM: And (laughing) they are temporarily insane.

SF: (Joining in) Yes!

JM: Whereas, if you get comfortable with leaving your ego aside—because there are many times when you don't need an ego, right?

SF: Ah. . .I'm already detached—let me tell you! I feel like I'm dangling out in space all alone—I have to tell you—most of the time.

JM: And so you experiment with—when don't you really need an ego—and you decide—okay, you know, I'll drop it, I'll let it go, That might be, for me, when I'm composing; certainly that would be a time when it would be (artistically) suicidal to try to stay inside my "Joseph" – or while I'm in the middle of a lake doing a long distance swim—why should I bother having a "Joseph"?

SF: Right. . .

JM: And more and more, as you experiment with it, you find that you can be free of that self even when you're among people—you can be standing, looking at, talking to somebody—and they may be thinking you have a self there, whereas, from within yourself, you are beholding the same situation from your 'eternal eye'—or your 'eternal I', however you may wish to describe it.

SF: Absolutely.

JM: And that's okay, that's fine—and there's nothing wrong in that.

SF: Oh. . .

JM: But I promise you—unless you have neurological damage or some temporary organic problem, you will always have your self in your back pocket when you need it; you're not going to wind up in a mental ward somewhere!

SF: No, I don't feel that way at all, and if anything, I'll just walk away from earthly 'everything' and enter into the void, because that's where I want to go right now.

JM: If you like to read and you find that the resonance of other people can provide some peace for you, I highly recommend the books of Bernadette Roberts, who was a Catholic nun, and whose interior reflective process ultimately led to the dissolution of her sense of self—and who had get accustomed to a new life without a self—and she was the mother of four! — because she felt as if her self was actually suddenly taken from her, much more radically than I think you are describing.

SF: Well, but I dream of such, I feel like that's actually living inside me, that I could do that, but I also feel compelled to—well, this is the great struggle—to stay with Patrick and to evolve with the earth's evolution in a kind of outer way, because there've been moments when I've wanted to give up on the earth itself and just drop out, so I could 'drop in'.

JM: Well, that usually doesn't happen even when people think it's happening because the life impulse is so strong—

SF: Yes—

JM: I don't know what your meditative background is,

but I've tried and done everything from the crown chakra down; for many years, because I was a little too ardent at performing kriya meditation, my initial out-of-the-body experiences destabilized and disoriented my nervous system. I thought I wanted the state you described when I was studying in Bologna Italy as part of my music curriculum in 1969, and my kriya practice was informed by the intensity that caused me to say to my academic mentor on the trip, "If I don't have a spiritual experience this year while I'm in Italy, I'm going to kill myself," —a rather strange, hyperbolic statement—since I know I wasn't about to do that, but it shows how strongly I longed for such an experience.

SF: Oh my God! (laughing)

JM: So I left the *pensione*—a kind of hostel or hotel— where everybody was too close around me—all the other students—and I got a bike and found a chalet just off of Via San luca, halfway up the side of a mountain at the top of which was the church San Luca – Saint Luke's – itself. Across the road from the hillside residence from who I rented a tiny villa was a convent of nuns that had been rescued from the Nazis by American soldiers in the Second World War; they were very kind to this young American – myself – who lived on the farm across the road from them. I'm not sure – perhaps they were praying for me – or maybe it was the spiritual energy harbored in San Luca – all I know is that I would perform massive amounts of Kriya meditation on the crown chakra practice of the internal sound that Patrick and I were talking about, and I would be lifted out of my body while my body was sleeping, in the middle of the night, and subjected to very high-frequency energies, which, aside from stressing my system, intrigued me explore further on, until one night I found myself out of my body again, and racing through deep space toward what seemed to me to be the Center of all Being – a vast, limitless Light; and I knew intuitively that when my being hit that Light that I would not die, but that all that I knew to be my human self would dissolve, that I would no longer be Joseph—I would be another form of universal being—and at that point only, Stephanie, did I realize that I very much wanted – because I was only 21—that I very much wanted my human-level life—

SF: Yes—

JM: I wanted my family, I wanted my friends, I wanted my life on earth, I wanted to have adventures, I wanted to write music, I didn't want to end the story and return to the Universal prematurely. And I felt, "Oh my God, this Power is so strong, and I'm going to plunge into it in a moment – there's no way that I can turn around. But I have to tell you that the Godhead – or whatever you wish to call that Source – is a respecter of human will, that nothing, as Edgar Cayce said, is senior to the human will – which is a strange thing to believe, but that's the whole purpose of life – we are given choice, and we can choose the way we want to go – and the moment I knew that I wanted my life, I remember cringing away from the Light and bracing all the 'muscles' of my being to put on the brakes, so to speak, I found myself thudding back into my body, covered with sweat, my heart beating seemingly hundreds of times per minute – almost like a psycho-spiritual crash landing. Now, that was an experience that forever erased any doubts or questions about the continuity of life, and the sanctity of life — but it also — because it was a forced experience — burnt out my neurological wiring for a very long time.

SF: Yes, I want to tell you that this is the same experience — but without my intention — that I had *kundalini* (activation of the evolutionary life-force within the spinal column) rising involuntarily from the age of — well — maybe 12 all the way to — it stopped at 20 or 21. I had no idea what it was, but it was always a near-death because I was going into the Light and my body was completely vibrating and I had no ability to move; and there was a roar with it—I didn't learn what it was 'til I was 18. It was terrifying. And I would stop it just as I was going to go into the full Light.

JM: Yep—well, then, you have a very early and intimate understanding of what is going on.

SF: I haven't linked it to what was going with me — because you're, like, completely re-wiring my brain: I certainly haven't thought about this silent sound that I'm hearing as relating to the kundalini, but now that I think about it – and if I put them together – it becomes a positive experience.

JM: Well—the *kundalini*—you won't keep getting that experience because once it becomes opened, it becomes an active state of being; I'm assuming that might be the case with you.

SF: Well, I was on the spiritual path my whole life, really, but from leaving home on, it was climbing the mountain; but I always think—if I could conjure *kundalini* and perhaps navigate it rather than have it take over. . .

JM: Before we go on – is what I'm saying meaningful to you?

SF: *Very!* – oh my God, completely and utterly. . .

JM: Okay then – may I finish my little adventure then, so you can see how I managed to stay on earth! Because, after that experience, I was virtually an empty shell for many months. . .and I felt no emotion, I felt no desire to eat or to do anything in particular. Music had no more meaning for me—if you can understand that kind of 'burnt-out-ness';

SF: Wow!

JM: Everything I did had to be done by an act of will.

SF: Wow!

JM: And that's because I had violated the natural parameters through which a human being functions; I'm telling you this not to tell tall tales, but because whenever you force an experience there's a price to be paid –

Sf: Yes.

JM: And I paid that price; and I had my doubts at times

(about survival) but here I am, 45 years later, to tell you that I made it—and the way that I made it may be very seminal for you: some years prior to going to Italy I had read a book by the title of *Hara*—and Patrick may know about this –

PF: Yes –

JM: *Hara* is the Japanese word for the area of the pelvis and lower belly, and it is the center of life in the eastern world—China, Japan, Asian culture—it is the center of life energy – okay?

SF: Okay. . .

JM: That is where women conceive and is the center where the procreative energies dwell in men and women, the deeper pelvis – and it is where the best and deepest breath emerges from, and it is the place babies and people who aren't uptight breathe from. You've observed this, haven't you?

SF: Yes, mm hm.

JM: And you'll find that western people and most intellectual have haras—or lower bellies—which are tightly constricted or hard and inflexible. So, this is the only unprotected area of the body, this lower abdomen, it has no ribcage, it has no thorax, and only in that way can it always remain flexible and alive.

SF: Mm, wow.

JM: And if you look at the culture of the east, whether it's in the art of flower arranging, or the art of archery or the martial arts, there is a foundational practice of centering oneself in the hara, otherwise known as the *tantien* — the Field of the Elixir, or the Field of Life – and of doing everything from there. To phrase it in musical terms – let's say I was a singer, or even a speaker, and my voice was like this (*JM imitating a shallow, constricted, upper-throat/nasal voice*) and my voice was like and my voice was just coming from my throat and it was narrow and it wasn't rooted in reality; (allowing voice to expand into torso again) whereas if my voice is like this, it's coming through a whole-body voice — it's rooted in my legs, my guts, my chest, my torso-- even the earth. So everything we do, when it's 'earthed' and grounded, assumes much greater voltage and balance — can you see that?

SF: Yes — oh absolutely.

JM: So I read this book six ways from Sunday — *Hara, the Earth Center of Man* — and I corresponded with the German psychotherapist named Karlfried Graf von Durckheim, an internationally famous healer who had spent 16 years studying Zen in Japan, and who also had a center in a valley in the Black Forest just above Switzerland. And prior to my going to Italy he invited me to his center. And, after my experience in Italy, I thought, that will be my salvation, if I can make it there. And I hitchhiked up through Northern Italy and Switzerland into Germany, where he had a whole valley of related therapists and spiritual works and Aikido instructors who basically resonated this need of the intellectual western mind to reconnect itself to the earth center, and I learned, through breathing, through meditation, through Aikido, through even the practice of musical art—because I was a musican – because I was *already* connected to the higher realms— that's not the issue. You can be connected to the higher realms and be insane on the human level, because of your inability to bring that into manifestation down here.

SF: Aha. . .

JM: I'm sure many, many people in mental hospitals have probably had transcendent experiences, but who had very poor personality grounding, very poor ego-structure that couldn't handle that higher manifestation.

SF: Mm hm. . .mm hm. . .

JM: So if you had come across me prior to my developing my 'earth-connection', you would have found a very bright, intellectual, smart, spiritually savvy guy—but you would have found great imbalance energetically, you would have found great lack of grounding, you would have found me in danger of floating off into the stratosphere. Think of it—I was already an intellectual guy, I was a conservatory-trained musician, which requires an incredible amount of cognitive knowledge and learning, and I was into higher kriya meditation. This is all a lopsided recipe on the transcendent side. But a (truly) human being is somebody who can operate in the human earth-realm as well, and for that you need grounding, you need balancing. As one spiritual teacher put it, "Stop concerning yourself with becoming divine; become truly human and you will *be* divine!"

SF: Yes. . .

JM: I don't know where you stand in this spectrum, but it may be worthwhile to consider that, throughout your life, you may have unknowingly been magnifying the upper end of your frequency spectrum, and whether or not it would help you—if you *want* to be here—to begin to grow your root system more.

SF: Yes—my sacral is undefined in Human Design—if you know what Human Design is; it's like, undefined—I have to define it, and that's just the area you're talking about.

JM: And that's not lower—in the spiritual sense—at all.

SF: Uh huh. . .

JM: It would be—let's say you were writing music as I do – and you had the whole orchestra at your disposal—the parallel of being told, "Ah, you must meditate on your crown chakra and you must lift your life force into the Godhead," would be somebody coming to you and saying, "No, you can't use any lower pitches, you can't use any bassoons or double basses, you can't use any cellos or percussion, bass drums—this is all forbidden to you; well, you know what kind of a piece of music you're going to arrive at with those kinds of restrictions. . .

SF: Right, right. . .

JM: It's going to be very, very unnatural.

SF: Mm hm. . .

JM: So I've come to a new understanding and appreciation of our earthliness, of our lower vibrations—but not inferior vibrations; they are absolutely essential to our humanity, and for that reason I don't buy the version of awakening that the Hindus have evolved. I think that life on earth has an incredibly important purpose and that we're here for an incredibly important reason, and that we need to embrace earthliness and our life here in very lusty, gutsy ways—while we retain that higher frequency spectrum. That's where I've arrived, anyway, and we can talk more at some point about how I did that or how you might want to explore that if you think it's a ripe area for exploration.

SF: I do—and, I don't know—I've just been very humbled by this conversation and very grateful for it; it just comes on the tail of a humbling, awakening weekend that Pat and I have been having by ourselves, there's just such a sense of things changing on so many vibratory levels right now that are assisting all of us. It's been wonderful talking to you, and I feel I shouldn't take more time out of your conversation with Pat, and I look forward to speaking together again.

JM: Sure—just feel out how you feel about what we've shared, and if you want to speak further, that's fine.

SF: Alright, wonderful—well, here's Patrick—thank you, Joseph.

JM: Sure. . Bye-bye. . .

PF: Wow, that was beautiful, Joseph. What a wonderful dissertation—I loved it very much; and I'm familiar with all the terms and everything used. I've been doing lower abdominal breathing for a long time. Years ago, in 1974, when I was in Los Angeles, a Korean qigong master came who was demonstrating some things—he could take a one inch iron bar, and he'd hold in both his hands – one hand on each end, and he'd put his chi into it and it would turn into rubber, and he'd wind it in a circle. And then no one, of course, could straighten it back out again; he did things like this, so I went to see him, and he told me that he was from a monastery in the mountains of Korea where the master was 300 years old, and he did a thing called gold needle acupuncture, where you take pure 24 carat gold needles and you insert them permanently into the body,; and they don't migrate because they're 24-carat soft gold, and your body forms scar tissue around them and that holds them in place. If they were hard needles they'd migrate and kill you. So I underwent a period of 6 weeks in which he put 128 gold needles in my body, up and down my spine and all over my body. And he said my chi meridians were the size of your little finger; he said that in a few years my meridians would be the

equivalent of a meter in diameter. And then he said —
in 15 years you're going to need to have all these gold
needles put in your head, and I said "Where will you
be in 15 years?" And he said, "I'll probably be back in
the monastery in Korea," – and by the way he was a
Korean national martial arts champion—and he had
told me he was walking in the hills one day and he saw
some bandits attacking an old man; and he was
running to rescue the old man when he saw the old
man put his palm out and one of the bandits fell down
dead—he didn't touch the bandit – and when this man
examined the bandit's body, all the bones in his chest
were crushed. So he said to the master, "Would you
please teach me your art?" and so he took him as a
student. But anyway, going back to this – that was in
1974 he put the gold needles in me and, exactly 15
years later—I'm living in Sedona, Arizona—and a 93-
year-old Japanese surgeon heard of my products and
wanted to come visit me, and I said okay – that was in
August in 1989—15 years later; and he came and he
said he was an acupuncturist and a surgeon, and I said
I had all these gold needles in my body and all that,
and the surgeon looked at me and he said "I studied
gold needle acupuncture at a monastery in Korea
where the headmaster is 300 years old. And he felt the
gold needles in my body and everything, and he said,
"When is your birthday?" And I said "October 11th."
And he said, "I will go home to Japan, get the gold
needles, and on your birthday I will complete the gold
needle acupuncture. " And so, on my birthday,
October 11, 1989, he came back, and he put 120 gold
needles in acupuncture points in my head—and so

now I have 256 gold needle acupuncture points in my body. Who can figure this? When I'm 17 years old, I'm a self-trained gymnast, because my school back then in Houston—Belair—Texas, didn't have any gymnastic program—and I had injured myself—dramatically – because I didn't have a teacher, but I became a world class gymnast. But anyway, I'm training in the gym in the YMCA, and I see this guy in white robes and a turban, and a beard, walking across the gym with his eyes on me – and glides across the gym and said to me, "Are you Patrick Flanagan?" And I said, "Yes," and he said, "I've come from India to teach you a mantra, and I have to back to India tomorrow, so will you please come with me to my hotel room—I have to teach you this mantra." So I went with him to his hotel room, and he had a little kitchenette hotel room, and he taught me the mantra, and then he taught me how to cook some Indian dishes with cumin and other Indian spices. Then he said, 'Now do this mantra—and 'I'm leaving for India,' and I said, "Well, how do I get a hold of you?" and he said, "You don't." And I said, "Well, what happens next?" And he said, "If you need more instructions someone will come from India and give them to you." And I said, "Well, how will they find me?" and he said, "They will find you"—and he left. It wasn't until 3 months ago I heard about this guy Babaji, and there was a film of him in 1980 and he only came in for like, 3 years and then he died. And when I saw the picture of him—he was the guy that came in from India in 1962. And the mantra was very strange because it was a combination of two mantras—it was a Krishna mantra and a Shiva mantra combined together. And when I've told some people who were not mystics, but just from India, they said, "Well, oh no, that can't be, because, you know, it's not done." And then several months ago a guy came who was in a Hari Krishna temple for 30 years who had studied Sanskrit, and I told him the mantra, and he said that because the Shiva mantra is "Om navashivaya" and the Krishna mantra is 'Hari Om'—okay —and what he had given me was, "Hari Om Nam Om Shivaya", and not "Nama shivaya" but "Nam Om Shivaya"; and the guy I had talked to said, "Nam Om and Nama" are the same thing; they can be used interchangeably. And so, the way he gave it to me, I had to chant it very loud and resonate it through my sinuses and my whole body, and it goes like this: *"Hari Om Nam Om Shivaya"* —like that. And anyway, these stories go on and on – I've raised cobras, I smoked cobra venom, which is a Shivite practice in India—my whole life is full of magical things like this.

JM: Did you find the practice of that new mantra a fruitful practice?

PF: Oh my God, yeah! What happened, is, right after that I entered my first gymnastics competition, which happened to be the AAU Southern United States Gymnastics Championships, and there were people competing who were going to be in the Olympics in Mexico City in a few years from then; and what happened is that I went in and they said "Well, you've never competed before so you have to come in as a novice; if you do well there, you could compete as an intermediate," and if you did well there you could go into the senior championships. And what happened is that I competed as a novice gymnast, and I won every gold medal that there was in every category, and they said "Well, if you have enough energy tomorrow, you can enter the intermediates; and so what happened was I went into the intermediates the next day – it was on Saturday – and I won every sing gold medal in every category in the intermediates. They said, "Well, I know you've competed 2 days running, but if you have enough energy, you can enter the senior competition on Sunday." What happened is, I was weak, I couldn't even hold a handstand; I did my mantra for 2 hours that night – and did it laying down, because it would resonate my whole body. And I went in on Sunday and entered the senior competition, and I won every single gold medal against Olympic gymnasts and everyone in the senior competition. And then they said, "We'd like you to go to the Olympics in Mexico City." In the meantime—my mother thought I was gay—for whatever reason—and she talked to the draft board and wanted to draft me into Vietnam in order to make a man out of me. So I met this girl in psychology class who I liked a lot, and we had a date, and during our date we told each other how our families were controlling us, and we decided to get married to get away from our families. And the following Saturday, one week later we got married, much to the relief of our families, and we were married for 11 years, and she's the mother of my two children.

JM: Was that Gael?

PF: No—Gael was my fourth wife—I've had four wives legally, and Stephanie is my fifth; and ours is a spiritual marriage. In the palm of my hand I have four wives, and it says that my fourth marriage would be a long marriage and she would die, and that was Gael; Gael and I and we were married for 14 years and she died. And Stephanie and I have been together for 16 years now. But it got my mother off my back, and I didn't get drafted to Vietnam. My mother, in many ways, was evil and was doing her best to destroy me, and did things to me that no mother should ever do to a child, and it's made me multiple ways —Stephanie has said to me from the things that my mother did to me, she is absolutely surprised that I'm not gay, because – horrific things, is all that I can say, but that's another story.

JM: Coming back around for a moment to your first book —as I read *Pyramid Power*, I see the mind of an individual who is about as far from a writer as I am from a scientist, and who is much elemental and scientific in his thinking—you're language is the language of a man who is defining facts and trying to establish principles—but which is not exactly user— friendly for ordinary mortals.

PF: Well, I have to tell you something—I've worked Dr. Dwight who was an information specialist, professor of Physics at Harvard and then Tufts University; and he was my partner when we did dolphin research for the Naval Ordinance Testing Center—the Navy—and Wayne Bateau had something he called 'ventilated prose' – and I wrote the book in ventilated prose. In a sentence the spacing was one space and between paragraphs it was three spaces; and between sentences it was two spaces. And each sentence had its own surrounding space, and it was laid out in such a way—what I tried to do was make each sentence so important that it was self—contained, with no extraneous stuff in there. And the result of that was that, over the years, I have so many compliments from people on the ventilated prose—and that might be one reason why the book took off and sold a million and a half copies —because no book sells a million and a half copies like that – self—published—and making enough money that I was able to stop consulting and stop working for the government. And I've had, over the years, so many compliments on the layout of that book and the ventilated prose that you can't even begin to believe it. And true, I'm not a writer—but, just the layout and presentation of that book—

JM: Right—no—if you're going to write about 'hard' science as you were trying to do there, you've got to ventilate it and provide 'white space' for the brain to absorb that.

PF: Right.

JM: So in spite of its distilled wisdom, it was received well by the public.

PF: Yes.

JM: And as I recall, you followed that with *Beyond Pyramid Power*?

PF: I did, and *Beyond Pyramid Power* was extremely successful—not as successful as *Pyramid Power*; I mean, *Pyramid Power* launched the entire pyramid revolution in the *world*; people started building and meditating and living in pyramids because of that book—building pyramidal buildings in Las Vegas – and in Russia, the Russian pyramids—the people in Russian who are the principle pyramid people have acknowledged me as being the reason why they started building pyramids in Russia.

JM: Well, I think I must have been one of the first purchasers of your frame—wood, plastic—canopy pyramids

PF: (Chuckles hard)

JM: And also, something I lost—I'd love to have a replacement—you had a 2—dimensional pyramid disc –

PF: Yeah – called the 'sensor' —

JM: —which I used to wear religiously; people always used to ask me what it was. And I thought that was a lovely idea, provided you actually could somehow collapse those energies to be functional even on a 2-dimensional surface.

PF: Not only did that happen, but Professor Callahan at the University of Florida, Gainesville, had this infrared spectrometer that would detect energies in the range of 1 millimeter through a 25 millimeter wavelength—it was then called the XM and is now called the Terraherz Band—I had this pyramid grid that had these little 1-inch pyramids, and he took it down, and we found out that, when you blow air over the grid, it produces all these wavelengths in that band. Not only that, but then he took my sensor—the flat pyramid—and he put that in his machine, and it was producing the same wavelengths as the pyramid.

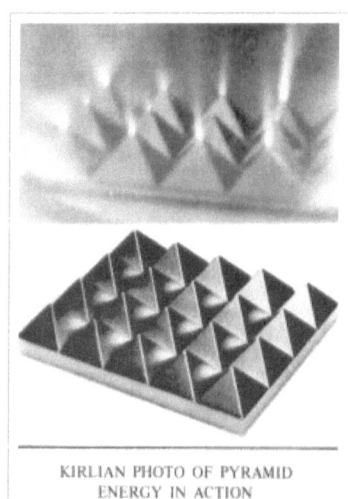

KIRLIAN PHOTO OF PYRAMID
ENERGY IN ACTION

JM: Wow. Well, I have no trouble believing that, because as I'm speaking to you right now, I'm sitting under one of Nick Edwards' 9-pyramid grids—and I have three of them, and this one is right over my musical workspace—and I have not ceased to feel it since I sat here to call you; and this has been hear for 3 years.

PF: Yes –

JM: And this is nothing more than an expansion on your mini—pyramid grid design.

PF: Yes, that's exactly what it is.

JM: So, what I really think is that, on a soul level, you've really inspired the soul of Nicholas to produce—

PF: Oh, absolutely, yeah—

JM: —such high quality.

PF: Yes, and not only that, but on the Giza plateau, where the Great Pyramid is built, there's always a 5 to 10 mile per hour breeze that's blowing—always—and one of the things is that that wind blowing across the pyramid generates these vortices that amplify the pyramid's power. And so, if you had a computer fan or something blowing air through those pyramids, it would amplify the effect.

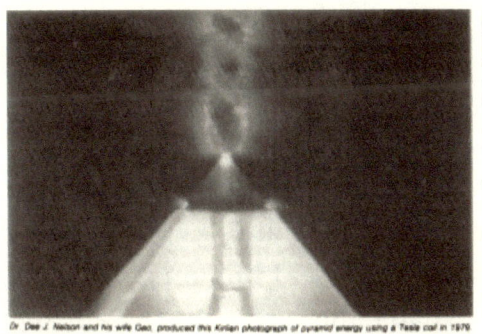

Dr. Dee J. Nelson and his wife Geo. produced this Kirlian photograph of pyramid energy using a Tesla coil in 1979

Dee J. Nelson and his wife Geo produced this Kirlian photograph of pyramid energy using a Tesla Coil in 1979.

JM: Is the effect to be found in the blown air, or at the

sight of the blowing

PF: No, the effect is the air blowing and vibrating across the pyramid structure itself, forming these vortices around the structure.

JM: So they stay in place—like standing waves?

PF: Yes.

JM: Wow – I'm going to try that today; I think Radio Shack has these little fans.

PF: Oh yeah – they do. And you get one that isn't noisy so it doesn't bother your consciousness to have that sound in the background.

JM: Nick (Edwards) just recently spoke to me about a whole slew of inspirations that I guess came through his reconnection with you –

PF: Yes.

JM:--including something a little more apartment—worthy, along the lines of the vertical Russian design?

PF: Yes, as a matter of fact, he's going to call that the Pat Flanagan Pyramid, and we're going to manufacture them, and I sent him one of the original sensors like you had—the disc – and I sent him my latest one, which is called the sensor V, which is something I made recently, and he's taking that to the injection moulder, and the injection moulder is going to create those, and we're going to put them on top of the Patrick Flanagan Russian Pyramid, and you can take that off the pyramid and hang it around your neck and energize your body.

JM: I think that's a brilliant idea; so it's going to be virtually the same sort of device as his treatment dish (a small disc—platform that plugs into one Edwards' pyramid connectors)

PF: And not only that—we have them in gold—plated, cast with multi—layers of metal that have an Orgone effect, and we sell those for $680, retail, and so Nick is going to sell those, and we're also going to have the treatment disc as well as the Patrick Flanagan Pyramids—it's all coming together beautifully. You know, the Russian pyramids, mathematically, are directly related to the Great Pyramid. Mathematically, they're perfectly related. I could send you the math on it and show you what it is.

JM: That would be fine; but if you could translate it into terms that were understandable on the practical level – do you feel that the effects are appreciably different than what people purvey as the pyramid based on the Cheops dimensions?

PF: Yes, well, they're both Golden Ratio angles; in fact, the Russian pyramid is actually a more perfect Golden Ratio pyramid than the Cheops. They're both Golden Ratio pyramids, but it's amazing that—one thing—in Russia they've published hundreds of scientific papers on the Russian pyramids, and, just to give you one example, they measure the power of antibiotic by how much killing effect it has on bacteria; and what they did was, they took this antibiotic and put in a Russian pyramid for one month, and then they tested it—and they could dilute it a million times, and even at a dilution of one millionth it had the same bacteria killing power as the original.

JM: So, it's almost like a homeopathic effect?

PF: Yes, you could dilute it homeopathically and have the same bacteria killing power as the original. If you took the original (untreated antibiotic) and diluted it one million times, it had no power. But what's treated in the Russian pyramid—that's just one Russian scientific paper. In Russia there's a man by the name of Goland who spent $500,000,000 building those Russian pyramids all over Russia, and in places where he built them, flowers started popping out of the ground that were considered to be extinct a million years ago.

JM: Really!

PF: Yes, and they're growing around all over the pyramid.

JM: So, you're quite willing to grant validity to what I've read – that the vortices coming off these structures are either palpable or functional even at the levels of air flight paths above the earth?

PF: Oh, absolutely. But it's not the air vortices, it's that the air flowing across is amplifying what's called the torsion field of the pyramid. There's a whole thing in Russia that the torsion field was actually a third force;

you know, you have electricity, magnetism and gravitation, and the torsion field is another force that makes everything work. In fact, the torsion field is a twist field—it's what gives DNA its twist, it what makes the spiral galaxies spiral, and the mathematics of the spiral are all Golden Ratio – they're all Fibonacci—which is the mathematics of the Great Pyramid and the mathematics of the Russian pyramids; and it's also the mathematics of the pyramids in Mexico.

JM: This is wonderful stuff; so this is a whole new chapter in both your lives—

PF: Oh, absolutely. Yeah—no—Nick and I, it's amazing—I have such respect for Nick and the pyramids he's made, and now the pyramids we're creating together. It's awesome—I'm sitting here looking at them now.

JM: It's beautiful—because, if you weren't looking closely, you would mistake Nick for a retired cowboy—

PF: (Laughs hard)

JM: —Kind of a laconic, not to given to too much intellectual discourse—and yet, when he opens up, he starts talking real esoterica.

PF: Oh yeah—exactly. Nick is as humble, beautiful spiritual man who you have pull out these things out of him, but once you start pulling them out, you realize how amazing he is.

JM: And he's very funny as well.

PF: Yeah—my experience is that I can't make it through life without a sense of humor.

JM: So this brings us back to your youthful antics. . .So you contacted him, and he obviously responded. .

PF: Yes.

JM: And what were given to tell him? Why did you contact him?

PF: Well, he was already aware of me and my stuff, but someone told me about a dentist treating dental implants in pyramids. . .

JM: So this had to be some years after you had written Pyramid Power, because Nick had to have time to learn how to do this and to produce his products.

PF: Right. I'd say it was maybe 4 years after I wrote *Pyramid Power*.

JM: Was he excited to meet you?

PF: Yes—he was. At first there was a little bit of a challenge, because we were basically in competition with each other—he's selling pyramids and I'm selling pyramids, you know. But the thing is, I was so impressed with what he was doing I had to meet him; and we met each other and got to know each other, and we hung around. .

JM: How old would you have been?

PF: Let's see, I wrote *Pyramid Power* in 1972, so I would have been 28 years old, so we would have met when I was in my early 30's.

JM: So was it basically a collegial relationship—or did it turn into a friendship?

PF: First it was collegial, and then it turned into a friendship; I mean, we weren't close friends, but we hung around together. I had a Lincoln Mark IV—I don't remember what he was driving—and we'd go somewhere and we'd kind of race each other all over town (laughing)

JM: So you were both still feeling your oats. . .

PF: Yeah, sure; from Glendale I moved over to these big towers in Marina del Rey; anyway, he was in Burbank at the time.

JM: And this was all that you did—you never held other positions?

PF: He made his products and you did your research and sold your products. And he never sold my products and I never sold his products. What happened is that I had a partner in my business—his name was Duke Lanfre—and we had a company together called Pyramid Products—and Duke and I had a falling out, and what happened is that Duke had intended for his son to take over the business, but his son was kind of like the little rich boy who wasn't tuned in, so Duke ended up giving the business to Nick, unbeknownst to me – so that's kind of where that went.

JM: So there was no resentment there on behalf of Nick?

PF: No, I had no idea—Nick only told me recently that Duke had given him the business. He was unable to get those little 1-inch pyramid grids which had 15 pyramids—so the pyramid grid that you've got there from Nick is kind of like Nick's version of that. In my book, *Pyramid Power*, there's a picture of those pyramid grids with energy coming off the top.

JM: Yes—and that brings up a whole issue I wanted to ask you about: I know that the Kirlian phenomenon is used by almost everybody as a justification for the effectiveness of their energy tools, and yet I've read fairly scholarly criticisms saying that is far from an indicator of any kind of dynamic energy. What's your feeling of Kirlian as a way of testing or proving energy?

PF: Well, a Russian scientist—Karatka, I believe—developed what's called the GDV machine, which is the Kirlian device into which you place your fingers, and that makes a snapshot of the Kirlian discharge of each finger, and based on that the computer analyzes it and tells you what organs of your body are out of balance; and it's beem well recognized and used as a medical diagnostic device all over the world.

JM: So it does reflect valid energy emanations from the body?

PF: Yes it does, mm hm.

JM: And it is the case that the brighter or whiter the readout or glow, the higher the energy field.

PF: Not necessarily; it can mean that you're losing energy. You know, my experience now is that I can see auras and developed that ability when I was 30 years old—actually I developed that ability when I was a kid, and it got turned off and turned back on again—and so I always thought the bigger the aura the more powerful the person was; and then I met a Sufi master from Istanbul who had no aura. And I thought, 'How can he be a master? He has no aura.' but what he was doing was—he wasn't just spinning his energy out all over the place, radiating it out; he collapsed it, so that all of his energy was self-contained, and he would release that energy consciously when he wanted to heal someone or do something. And I'm now of the opinion that the brighter and the whiter the Kirlian photo may be doesn't necessarily indicate that the person has more energy, because if it was a perfectly tuned field all around in the balance—but coming off that field, if there are gaps in it—places where there is no emanation—that's because of an energy imbalance in the body.

JM: In your book, *Pyramid Power,* you have a photograph of a finger before and after—

PF: Well, the thing is—I discovered Kirlian photography before Kirlian—that's the point

JM: What is the effect on Kirlian when somebody sits

under the pyramid, then?

PF: If you use the GDE you might find that their energy becomes more balanced, and you may even find that it increases. The consciousness part of it is when we learn how to control our energies so we don't spend it, so you can control your energy and use it consciously—so there are two different things. Sitting under the pyramid, one of the first things we noticed, if you use an EEG machine, we found out that when people sit under the pyramids they start producing a lot of really strong alpha waves. But if you start using my Neuroophone, the person starts producing waves like he's meditated in a cave for 30 years—so these things are all related.

JM: But in general, do you feel the pyramid lends an energy enhancement

PF: Yes—oh, definitely. Definitely it's an energy enhancement.

JM: Whatever the Kirlian particulars are, you feel there's a consistent, reliable effect from the pyramid?

PF: Yes.

JM: And have you ever taken time to research cone energy?

PF: Oh I have, of course. In my book, *Beyond Pyramid Power*, I talk about cones. In fact, if you have a pyramid with four sides and you make one with 8 sides, you have an octamid, and if you make one with

5 sides it's a pentamid. A cone is a pyramid with an infinite number of sides, and a cone at the right angles—that is, the angle of the Great Pyramid—it has the same power as the Great Pyramid, and you don't need to worry about orienting it to the earth's magnetic field. So a cone is a pyramid with an infinite number of sides, and if it's got the right angles, it's *extremely* powerful. That's why teepees—you know Black Elk who was friends with Crazy Horse and sitting bull—Black Elk said that when the white man took away their round houses, he took away their power; the earth is round, the sun is round, the moon is round, and that power comes from the round structure, and when the white man put them in square houses, he took away their power.

JM: It also might refer—I don't know how familiar you are with this – I've written extensively on it, and I know the gentleman who rediscovered it—it's called 'earthing'—

PF: Of course, yes, I was doing earthing in 1974—

JM: —where I'm sure the native Americans in their teepees were almost certainly in a situation where they were earthed, whereas the conditions within houses, with their floor structures, were almost never earthed situations.

PF: Yes, of course.

JM: And you're aware now that there are products that reconnect you to ground?

PF: Yes, I'm totally familiar with them; the thing is that you could have a square house with a dirt floor and it's not the same as having a pyramid or a teepee with a dirt floor.

JM: Oh, granted—I totally believe you. So, theoretically, a conical structure could be exponentially stronger than a pyramid.

PF: Oh, absolutely.

JM: Then what would prevent you and Nick Edwards from producing together some cones of various sizes.

PF: Nothing. We don't need to; the thing is, in my book *Beyond Pyramid Power*, I show how to make cones, you take a flat round circle and you cut a section out of it and then you bring that together in the form of a cone.

JM: So, does the angle matter greatly?

PF: Yes, totally. And it turns out—I've examined a lot of Indian teepees—and there's just a ratio, aesthetically, that the correct angle for a teepee cone/pyramid they've pretty much made them pretty much like the Russian angle.

JM: So then, pretty steep. . .

PF: Yes, because if they're flat and they're low, the poles tend to collapse, it tends to fall down, and if you make it a little steeper, they tend to remain stable.

JM: So in both cases—it doesn't matter—pyramid or

cone—is it your feeling—I know Nick Edwards is of the opinion his titanium frame pyramids are acting as antennas, much like modern radio antennas, whereas, I'm not sure that the major proportion of the energy isn't being conducted up from the earth rather than down from the atmosphere...

PF: It's hard to separate it, but I think that pyramids would work just fine in space.

JM: So they *are* like antennas.

PF: Yes—but the thing is that there's still a question of whether or not if those tubes were made out of aluminum or steel versus titanium—I believe that titanium has a much higher energy level, crystalline-wise, than other metals; that said, you can make a steel pyramid, you can make an aluminum pyramid, and they still have effects.

JM: Does enclosure make a difference?—because there are people who have built pyramid homes, you know.

PF: Well—yah!—they built pyramid homes after reading my book, you know.

JM: Are they any more valid or energetically intense than a pyramid frame of the same size.

PF: No—the thing is—there's a guy up between Chicago and Wisconsin, and he read my book and he's a builder, and he started building a pyramid house 10,000 square foot base, and he built the frame and everything, and then he covered it, and then he started making gold shingles—he'd take aluminum and gold plate it it, and they were like shingles, and he started covering it with gold, real 24—carat gold—plated, and when he was almost done, a natural spring came out of the ground dead—center under the pyramid and he had to tap it off, and it had so much water that he built a moat around the pyramid with a drawbridge. And still he had so much water that he made a lake; and then he started selling the pyramid water – and the whole thing was because that Pyramid Power pulled that water right out of the ground.

JM: That's astonishing—so this is still happening?

PF: As far as I know—I haven't talked to the guy for years—I can't even remember his name right now.

JM: Because people have written some fairly interesting books—Ed Petit and Bill Schulze—which have a lot of anecdotes in them—particularly a fellow up in Canada who would use them for people who would come to him for help with their health— remarkable stories about turning around children with behavioral disorders and all sorts of stuff, so it seems to me still a largely untapped area.

PF: It is.

PF: We weren't in contact from 1978 'til we met again Chichen Itza—

JM: What was that reunion like?

PF: Oh it was awesome, it was wonderful; and, of

course, by then we were communicating, and maybe a year and a half ago I had bought a Tesla Coil from Nick, and my Tesla coil burned out because it couldn't handle what I was doing with it. I'm driving to Los Angeles this weekend to the Consciousness Expo, and Nick and I have a booth together.

JM: What were you using the Tesla coil for, in your case?

PF: I was experimenting with it; Nick had one of his pyramids on top of it, and I was playing with it, and I have these other structures I built, playing with energy, we call it torsion field. The pyramid actually emits torsion field energy—but basically it's the energy of time—time itself is a torsion field.

JM: It's an intriguing concept. In my layman's mind, could I conceive this as the momentum of energy that occurs when space curves?

PF: Exactly! There's no such thing as a straight line, and a curve is a torsion field, and that's what makes the galaxies curve, and – you know, the planets don't roll around the sun in an ellipse, the planets travel behind the sun as it moves through space in a spiral—torsion manner and it's that energy that makes the whole universe run, and it's all Golden Ration, and it's all the same energy and the same mathematics used pyramids.

JM: This is fascinating, because in this paradigm you're describing, the shortest distance between two points is a curved line—it's like in Aikido or any martial art movement, when you want to generate the most energy, the most *ki*, you do it by moving along the lines of a spiral—

PF: Absolutely—yah!

JM: And that creates a momentum that can't even be equaled by a blunt, straight approach—and I think that's true even at a metaphorical level, such as in human relationship; if I just say, "I love you", that's nowhere near as potent as if I take what seems like an elliptical course where I might say, "You know, when I'm with you, I really feel something special . ."

PF: Yes. . .

JM: It seems more indirect, but it's really more direct because by means of that 'ellipticality' I'm actually able to really connect with you.

PF: Yes. . .

JM: And therefore, it's more effective.

PF: Man—beautifully said—I love that. . .You know, when I was a kid, I came in with martial arts skilled that were from a past life, because, being a small, short kid who had polio when he was 9 years old, the bullies always would go after me, you know, and whenever a bully would really attack me with the intention of hurting me, and something within me would make the right moves and the bully would end up going through the air, landing on his head, on gravel, and his head would get cut open and he'd be bleeding all over the place—and it was always the case where their head would be cut open. I mean, in the school, when someone would attack me, I'd end up bending them over and hitting them in the ass and their head would hit the locker and their head would bleed – it was always. . . And in high school guys from the football team tried that on me and I ended up hurting the biggest football player in school badly, and then they left me alone—and this was before anyone spoke about karate or anything. I have to say though, that when I was 9 years old, my uncle Mickey, who was in World War II, had studied jiu jitsu, and he gave me a book on jiu jitsu, and I learned all the nerve points and pressure points just from reading the book. My father worked for Shell Oil Company, and the vice president from the company was at this company picinic—and I"m 11 years old by this time, and he says to me, "I hear you know judo," and I say, "I know a little bit," and he grabbed my hands and said, "Okay, what would you do now?" and I twisted his arms and threw him over my shoulder.

JM: (laughing)Ah—you were a dangerous kid!

PF: Yeah—and he wound up on the ground flat on his back with the air knocked out of him. And everyone was laughing—but it was all natural to me; yeah, I read the book and everything—I think jiu jitsu is one of the most dangerous arts there is, you know.

JM: So it wasn't just your pugnacious Irish ancestors – you got this from your karmic past. . .

73

INTERVIEW WITH PATRICK TIMPONE

PT: What kind of a diet do you eat? We're going to talk about antiaging and scientists and about really understanding how the body works. What kind of foods have you gravitated to over the years?

PF: Well, I was a pure vegan/vegetarian for 33 years and out and then at the end of that period—I guess it was the 2000—on January 1, 2000, I had a friend that was a eating raw meat--raw everything, and he was so impressed with the way he felt that he convinced me to on January first 2000 I had purchased a fillet mignon and I had it ground; and at about five in the morning after New Year's Eve party I got home and of and I put a raw egg into the meat and some spices, and I mixed it all up and decided to take one bite of it with a forkful, and I had decided that it was either get going to kill me or—I didn't know what would do to me, honestly, after being up a vegan for that long—but I ate it and my whole body went "Oh my God—thank you so much for the protein, and I consumed the rest of it and then went to bed, not knowing if I was going to wake up. But I woke up several hours later feeling wonderful, And so for one year I ate a lot of raw meat, and now I'm away from that pretty much. I'm pretty much of a multi-vore; I eat all kinds of food, depending on where we are in and what the available local food is. But it's really important to have antioxidants; it's very important to have protein.

There is wonderful protein pill called MAP—M-A-P,

and it's the perfect amino acid formula of eight amino acids that are so perfectly balanced that when you can take eight pills, it's equal to eating a kilo of beef and they're all vegetarian sources—and when you when you process the protein there is no residue left over—nothing that your body has to eliminate that's toxic, and even people who are on kidney dialysis content can take it and they don't have any problems because with it because they can't take any other source of protein. Meat has the amino acids, but there's so much leftover crap from the protein. I think it's important for us to have some kind protein even if you get a good source of vegetarian protein or something like that; I'm all for that, too.

The guy who developed MAP is amazing; the city map I just here is messenger amino I highly recommend it—you know, I'm for health and for people getting the best they can no matter where they can find it. It's pure amino acids that have been pressed into tablets—nothing else, no excipients This was developed by Dr. Luca Moretti—he's Italian, he's amazing. I don't know how old he is right now but when he was, I guess, about 60 he took a course of his own tablets. They are expensive but when you think about that the expense that they are, they don't cost that much; if you take a tablets and it's equal to the to the actual pure eight amino acids you get in a kilo of steak; then they're actually not that expensive.

Q: If somebody wanted to do a vegetarian lifestyle, could they get away with taking this supplement?

PT: Oh yes, MAP would absolutely do it.

When you did the raw meat for a year, did you did you feel any kind of animal—or different--vibration that was unpleasant to you?

PT: I do what I do what the Indians do—I would go into an alpha state and contact the spirit of the animal that died, and I would then beg forgiveness for consuming what I was consuming, and would, in my reality, get permission from the animal for the right to consume it, because I know I was a vegan/vegetarian for 33 years, because of my concern for the suffering of animals, and I was deeply, deeply into it, but I am certain point after that 33 year period, I felt so out of balance and so weak, because I didn't have essential the amino acids. I felt like I like my body was deteriorating—and it was—quite rapidly after after those 33 years. Although I experimented with eating everything I could. I also went out back to eating eggs at that time, and that helped a lot. But the animal farming of the chicken farms and the meat farms are so cruel and so terrible. That's one of the things I liked about South Americans where we travel is that they are so poor that they don't have these the meat farms things are more natural. I still contact the animal spirit if I'm consuming those things.

I am a Cherokee Indian, from my knowledge, the Cherokees—and all the Indians that –I don't know if all the Indians did that, but I do know that many of the medicine men would contact the spirit of the animal and the animal would actually give itself up for them. I really believe that with all my heart, and because survival on this planet isn't exactly—you know, were not in the Golden age yet, in which there are no predators and there are no victims from predators, and I sincerely believe that were coming into a golden age, in which lions and lambs will lay down together, and the lions won't eat the lambs—I really believe that with all my heart, and I'm so looking forward to that.

Our guest is the lovely and talented Dr. Patrick Flanagan this morning; at age 11 he developed a system to detect the flight-paths of missiles coming over to the government to do that. I'm glad you're on our side!

Thank you! (laughing) I published in the science fair when I was I guess it was 12—I'd love it; but I published for all the ICBM missiles firings in the US, and where they were fired from, and all this stuff in a science fair that I won. I was in study hall in the seventh grade, and the principal came on the loudspeaker and he said "Patrick Flanagan, come to my office immediately—the Pentagon is here." And I went to the principal's office and there was a 5-star general from the Pentagon who asked me how I knew all their secrets, and I told him that I had a little device I'd developed that told me, and they sent a whole team from Wright-Patterson Air Force Base down to Houston and they took my invention away and made my father sign a nondisclosure agreement on penalty of death and said that if I ever talked about the details of it to anyone but an authorized Pentagon official that my parents would never ever see me again. So it was taken very seriously.

PT: And what was this invention?

PF: I got this idea because I have been experimenting with ionized gases—plasmas, and I discovered that that ionized plasma emits certain frequencies and so it was an extremely low frequency radio locator detector that could detect and differentiate between an atomic bomb and an ICBM being fired, and I was able to radio-locate every test. Back then they were doing above ground atomic testing and the ICBM clearance, because they were developing all these things and I tuned into them, and the and so as far as I know my discovery is still being used; of course, it's been improved, no doubt, with computers. But that that was really what got their attention; and so I worked for the government as a teenager and when I reached 17 I drove all by myself from Houston Texas to Stamford Connecticut to a Pentagon think tank and consulted for them in the summer and that led to other things--communicating with dolphins for the Office of Naval Research—ONR—and China Lake, and I became very involved, and that kept me from going to Vietnam, because I consulting for the government during the Vietnam War on all kinds of things. I stopped doing that when I reached 28 years old. I am I wrote a book called *Pyramid Power*, and no one would publish it. They said no one would be interested. So I borrowed 5000 dollars and I published 5000 for one dollar each—5000 hardback copies of *Pyramid Power*, and it took off like crazy and I sold one and a half million copies over the next few years. And since I owned it. It made me independent I didn't have to consult for the government or anyone else anymore and became my own inventor-businessman selling my inventions.

We're republishing it; it's going to be published as an e-book on Amazon, and we haven't really changed it because it's still applicable today as it was back then. I got hundreds of thousands of letters from people who read pyramid power, and it changed their lives, and I think it's time for another generation of people to tune into it.

I think I've seen pictures of you with these big pyramids that you can sleep in.

PF: Well, you can. I had a partner, and his name was Nick Edwards, and he had these titanium alloy pyramids that he had developed, and he and I developed some more together and were selling them, but unfortunately Nick suffered some kind of aneurysm in his brain. One day he was perfectly healthy and the next day he was he was gone. We no longer sell pyramids on my website, but *Pyramid Power* will tell you how to make your own pyramids, and also yacht so it's pretty valid stuff.

PT: How did they build the pyramids—do we know?

PF: Nope. We don't.

PT: Probably government contractors!

PF: There is a scientist by the name of Davidovitz who has pretty much established-- They had giant granite blocks and King's chamber—that the pyramid stones are actually a form of concrete—that they actually poured them in place, and he's got a lot of proof on that that I subscribe. Except for the granite blocks—the granite blocks were cut and how they hauled granite blocks winning 70 tons apiece up and made the roof of the King's chamber in the great pyramid—I've I spent about 3 1/2 years in Egypt and gone there 34 times. It's really a very, very fascinating place. I wouldn't go today because I think it's too dangerous; the last time we went was I guess in the year 2000, and we had to have armed guards with machine guns on the buses with us, and I decided that because I was invited by Anwar Sadat—I knew. I the Sadat family well, and they were wonderful family—I was invited to go to Egypt by Anwar Sadat and be with them in this parade in which he was murdered; but I. was unable to go. Otherwise I might not be here. But I think Egypt is a fascinating place, but you know the world's getting crazy.

ON IODINE

By the way I take iodine I've been taking for 18 years, and I'm a strong advocate of iodine, especially with

Fukushima and everything that's happening right now. I haven't taken any lately, and there's kind of a flu going around where I'm at (Ecuador) My body's fighting it off, but I took 100 milligrams a day every day for 18 years; and since I've been traveling I've been lax at it, unfortunately. But with iodine—it's in all of your bodily fluids, and all our cells need iodine, but if you take it with an iodine cofactor, which is the vitamin niacin—non-flushing niacin—it's called no flush niacin—that's a cofactor that helps the body absorb and use it, The product I take is called Iodoral—I actually helped develop it and but I do highly recommend Cayce iodine—I think it's wonderful. If you take iodine where you have about one part per million in all your bodily fluids, that one part per million is your first line of defense against every virus and of course it helps protects that the thyroid against problems with the iodine 13, which is rolling around the world, north and south of the equator along with other nucleides from Fukushima. I can't go into detail on those because that's a big no-no; you can get yourself killed by a talking too much about those things.

PT: What is the connection of the no-flush niacin with the iodine?

PF: Well it's a cofactor; your body cannot absorb the iodine without the no-flush niacin. Along with with 100 mg of iodine I take about 500 mg of the no-flush niacin. If you take ordinary niacin it can be very uncomfortable because of the flush, but for the iodine absorption the no-flush niacin is the perfect cofactor to make sure that your body absorbs and utilizes the iodine in all your cells.

ON, MEGAHYDRATE, WATER AND DR. HENRI COANDA

PT: Would you tell us about what your Megahydrate is and how it works?

Well, when I was working at the Pentagon think tank, I worked with Dr. Henri Coanda. and Dr. Henri Coanda is known as the father of fluid dynamics, and he had over 500 patents on fluid dynamics. There is not a single jet airplane in the air today or a helicopter that does not use something called the Coanda effect in order to get the maximum air flow in the air amplification over the wing surfaces and aircraft surfaces, no matter whether they're moving wings, as in a helicopter, or non-moving, as in a jet airplane. Dr. Coanda was 78 years old when I was working for the Pentagon, and they were working on a torpedo that would go a hundred miles an hour underwater without creating a wake, based on his design.

His girlfriend was Gloria Swanson, the film star; they used to take me out to lunch every day as I was there alone—I was 17, and on his 78th birthday they had a big party for him. He was an amazing man—he was in amazing shape; he smoked Gauloise cigarettes together, one after the other, lighting one with the other all day long since he was eight years old. And here he was, 78, and he was a very robust strong man, a big man, and so I said 'I hope when I'm your age I'm in the shape you're in—and he said, "Patrick, when you're 78 years old, we'll talk about it." And it got a big laugh from everyone.

But after that he invited me into his office that in this think tank, and he said that he had studied all the places in the world where people live to be naturally over 100 years old while maintaining excellent health. One of those areas is called Hunzaland land in the Himalayas, another one was Vilcabamba, in Ecuador, another is a high Mountain Valley in Georgia, in Russia, and there are two more—one in Mongolia and I'm not placing that the fifth one right now, but Dr. Coanda had traveled to all those areas before the turn of the century, and he had determined that it was the water they consumed that was the secret of their longevity, not necessarily what they were eating, because they ate different things in different areas. He gave me all of this research on water at that time and said that he didn't know why the water did what it did but he figured I would figure it out and make it available. So I worked from the age of 17 'til I was in my 30s, and I finally developed a product called Crystal Energy, and these are little drops that you add to water that make ordinary drinking water exactly the same as the kind of water you find naturally from the glaciers in Hunzaland.

And so I put that out; at first I put out 10,000 bottles and just gave them away, and then suddenly everyone wanted to continue having them. They had amazing healing properties on me—I'm speaking for myself; I bad been a world-class gymnast when I was 17—self-trained, and because I was self-trained I had a lot of accidents, and when I was 30 I was so kind of crippled up from all my accidents that I could hardly walk. So I started consuming huge quantities of Crystal Energy and all my aches and pains went away, so that was kind of like that the birth of my first product. But after I had developed Crystal Energy I had always wondered what is the difference between cooked food, especially fresh raw juices that you drink immediately after you juice—versus cooked food and juices that you kept in the refrigerator for half an hour after you made the fresh juice that didn't have the 'oomph' that it had if you drank it immediately out. I discovered an Ion called negative ionized hydrogen, or the hydride ion, which up until that point in science was considered to be so elusive. It is an antioxidant, but so elusive that, though it's supposed to be present in the juice, after half an hour is no longer there. You have other antioxidants but not the negative ionized hydrogen, and that led me to develop the product we call Megahydrate, which is a storage vessel for the most primordial antioxidant in the universe—the negative hydrogen hydride ion. We proved through publications in peer-reviewed scientific journals that the hydride ion could actually exist in water for 12 or even 24 hours after you put it in water, and that it still had these powerful effects on the body if you had them in a special kind of water that was ion stabilized; and it turns out the crystal energy helped that, so I eventually developed the Megahydrate. We don't advertise it—it's sold basically by word-of-mouth. Some of our distributors advertise it, but it's been so successful—it's selling all over the world and it's my primary nutrient, because you know we all can't eat a pure raw diet of fresh organic food, and also we have so many challenges today with the ionized radiation from Fukushima and also with ourselves and our bodies being constantly attacked by free radicals. And this is the only free radical neutralizer or antioxidant that neutralizes free radicals and does not in itself *become* a free radical. So I've been taking that for the last 20 years or so and that's my staple—I'm just taking three of them right now while we're talking.

You can do more than one Megahydrate in the glass if you want—you can pony up on them if you want, especially if you're under stress if you are under a lot of stress. No matter what the source of the stress is, we need more because stress causes free radicals in the body and can lower our immune system. We need all the help we can get in today's world, especially with chemtrails and get all the other things that are salting us--weather engineering, as they call it. You can take the Megahydrate and the crystal energy together, something I highly recommend. Crystal Energy alone is an amazing thing; it's so wonderful because it makes the water you drink more closely resemble the water that surrounds our cells, and the water surrounding our cells is not the same as the water we drink. When you add Crystal Energy to the water it lowers the surface tension so that the water wets the cells more efficiently enabling more efficient communications of nutrients into the cell and toxins out of cells.

ON THE MYSTERIES OF THE HEART & CIRCULATION

PT: We had a doctor on the show, Dr. Thomas Cowan, an MD doing a lot of research and investigation into the heart, and that his conclusions—and many scientists agree over many years—is that the heart is not a pump—it's just a muscle—he describes how it works, with the electrical charge of the blood and the cells creating a differential that's responsible for pumping blood through the body, and how the body also makes these ancillary or collateral arteries to make sure that the heart gets blood. He says all these bypasses or really not needed because the heart is not going to depend on just four arteries. Do you think that's true?

PF: Yes, it's totally true. I studied that myself a long time ago; some hydraulic engineers, some 25 or 30 years ago studied the capillaries and said that even though the heart does put out a pretty good wallop of blood into the into the aorta it would be impossible for the heart to produce enough pressure to pump all the blood through all the capillaries in the body; there are micro-muscular contractions going on all the time within the muscles that help pump blood, and also there are ions—you also mentioned grounding: if you walk daily out barefoot upon the earth you absorb electrons from the earth, because the earth is negatively charged, and those also help with your antioxidant power; all of these things work together. And in Holland there's Dr. Gerald Pollock's—his discoveries on water are profound—how water forms these the zones in the capillaries and so forth, and how ions help move blood cells through the blood vessels. I studied the subject of zeta potential years ago, where we had a camera and photographed the blood vessels in the eyes and would be able to see the blood cells going through the capillaries in the eyes one by one; we also know that when –by the way mega hydrate helps to charge the blood cells with their natural negative charge so that the blood cells can go through the capillaries in single file, because when the blood gets clogged—we did a lot of the studies using dark-field microscopes with the unit dark-field condensers, and we were able to show that if you take the two capsules in the Megahydrate –you put them in the in three quarters of a glass of water, you stir it up and let it sit for a couple minutes and then you drink it, it so charges the red blood cells that all the clumping goes away and all the blood returns to a beautiful, natural state where the blood cells can actually pass through the capillaries.

ON EARTHING

PT: Dr. Cowan was saying that the sun, grounding and touch were key to this whole system working. I was wondering—being an Indian—do you think pure leather moccasins still allow you to ground while walking on the ground?

PF: I do I do You know there were some grounding shoes available for a while that were awesome, and I have sandals and shoes that have copper electrodes on your toes and on your heel with that then go through to the ground. That way you don't have to actually walk barefoot, but you're grounded all the time. Unfortunately, I guess they didn't sell that well because I don't think you're available anymore. But moccasins –yes, and you know, the Cherokee nation of Indians—I mean there's so much Indian lore about why the Indians did what they did, and they knew intuitively—they didn't necessarily know scientifically like we do today—but they knew intuitively that grounding was extremely important for health, because Indians, you know, after a long day's ride, would just lay down flat on the earth and ground their whole body It's all connected, and we're just relearning what they did.

ON THE METAPHYSICS OF EATING MEAT

PT: Do you know if, when the Indians did have meat— which I guess they did on special occasions—if they cooked it or not?

PF: Well, we do know that when the Indians would would kill a buffalo they would eat its heart raw, l and that the heart, you know, has so much power in it and they did eat a lot of meat raw; then they would do they would cure it, and would dry it, and eat jerky and things like that. I don't have any specific memories from my ancestral line other than that I have had visual images of its coming somewhere in my body— I don't know if it's from my DNA or what—but I think that they did eat a lot of it raw, although they did they did learn how to cook from the white man (laughing).

MORE ON MEGAHYDRATE

When you take Megahydrate into your body it releases negative ionized hydrogen gas hydrogen gas, and so sometimes when you burp the burp will change in frequency because hydrogen is less dense than helium even the helium from balloons that makes you talk like Donald Duck. That's part of how the healthy negative ionized hydrogen is absorbed into the portal vein when you take it: part of it is released in the form of a negative ionized gas, so that's natural. I have hydrogen burps all the time and it doesn't bother me— I'm just on losing a little bit of the hydrogen that should be going in my blood.

We get about 13 milligrams of negative ionized hydrogen with every capsule of Megahydrate, and that makes a huge difference in our bodies. We know now that the NADH— Nicotinamide adenine dinucleotidehydride—breaks down in our mitochondria and the hydrogen ions actually help to form adenosine triphosphate, ATP, which is the fuel that the body runs on. And so The H on the NAD is the hydride negative ion, and when your body uses that to make ATP, then the NAD becomes NAD+, which needs another negative ionized hydrogen to do the same cycle over and over; and so when you we're younger we have enzymes called dehydrogenase that actually makes negative ionized hydrogen in the body in order to make NADH. But as we get older our enzyme systems suffer and we need external sources of H minus, such as eating raw food, fresh raw juices or taking a young Megahydrate all: and I am I had my three morning like that point: when you know I wonder what I'd like to pick the date at any moment on airplane traveling because the amounts I'm 5 feet four and I would hundred 20 when I was your age and the but I I had a friend who was 63 the way to hundred 20 pounds and he's the guy that started eating raw meat and for the first time in his life he put on 40 pounds of solid muscle will meet with you and he was an athletic trainer so he had that's why I I tried to roll me when I was after 33 years of being a vacant idea I was so impressed with the way his health changed and how he put on solid muscle that that's why I did it.

I find that the young that the H minus actually is very profound, and of course I think that pine pollen is excellent. As we get older—I'm 71—we tend to lose our testosterone; if becomes balanced—we have plenty of it, but it's not free testosterone so it can't be used to make muscle. You can take various supplements such as Tribulus Terrestres.

ON CRYSTAL ENERGY & MAGNESIUM

Adding Crystal Energy to a water vortex device causes the amount of bubbles to double or triple; the bubbles get smaller and the Crystal Energy has as a lot of it of minerals that are good for the body. But I highly recommend that everyone take magnesium as a mineral supplement. II take about 600 mg of magnesium every day. I do not take a calcium supplement; when we get older that there's so much calcium in processed food and other foods that we don't really need calcium; we need magnesium because magnesium helps the bones to absorb calcium and also silica is in the bones and we get silica from crystal energy. Also, I recommend that you get some of those minerals from this great Salt Lake you know which I recommend that people us. Crystal Energy does have a lot of trace minerals in it, but the other thing is that if you if you drink any kind of natural herb tea that you get more usable minerals than you do from taking a lot of the inorganic minerals.

So I don't worry too much about minerals are I know that if you can get food that's grown in volcanic soil and where that the soil is been processed by biodynamic gardening and things like that you get you get so much nutrition from that kind of food.

PATRICK TIMPONE INTERVIEW: 2

SAFE & UNSAFE FOOD, CLEANSING THE BODY OF RADIATION

Unfortunately, Hawaii is extremely radioactive now and I don't recommend foods from Hawaii anymore.

I'm so sad about that. I use to live on Maui, near Haiku, and there is a restaurant—I don't want to name the name—that serves sashimi and rolled fish and such things, and we talked to the owner, who was a good friend, and he said that that they now have to cut cancerous tumors from the fish before they served it, because the waters there are so radioactive that the fish are just loaded with cancer. It's just a very sad state.

There's not really any way to directly clean up Fukushima—we have to clean ourselves up. I understand the Dr. Sircus came out with a lot of information all about sodium bicarbonate, and it turns out that sodium bicarbonate helps a lot with removing some of the radioactive isotopes. Also, MSM, organic sulfur, helps sulfate and remove the heavy metals from the body; and there've been some studies recently that showed that the zeolites to work as well as as some people were saying, but that definitely sodium bicarbonate, MSM, Megahydrate and Crystal Energy also help to clear heavy metals out of the body. I highly recommend organic sulphur, but since I'm traveling I can't carry a lot of it with me. The one thing that I miss the most is large quantities of that—I used to take about 3 tablespoons a day of organic sulphur. The thing about organic sulfur or MSM is that it can actually combine with the all the heavy elements-- except for iodine—and we don't want to chelate the iodine out of the body; but it does sulfate those heavy metals and help remove them from the body, and helps remove the fluoride from the pineal gland, and so does the sodium bicarbonate (baking soda). We can take a half a teaspoon to a teaspoon a day. Dr. Sircus recommends it in carbonated water.

I was fascinated by one of the studies that he told about in which they gave a large group of people sparkling water to drink for six months, after which they gave them still water for six months and then measured all their bodies' parameters—and it turned out that the sparkling water was extremely healthful in changing the LDL and HDL cholesterol ratios in a very highly positive way. I've always been attracted to natural sparkling water, especially as it comes out of the ground; and now I know why—because it contains euro bicarbonates, and that it turns our body needs carbonation in order for the oxygen to move efficiently in our cells and for the carbon dioxide is eliminated. A lot of people are deficient inCO_2; all this talk about the weather and the CO_2 cycle in nature have all been shown to be true—the more CO_2 the plants have, the better.

THE NEUROPHONE

I invented the Neurophone when I was 13. We didn't know how it worked, but the original Neurophone was gigantic—it covered maybe a 4' x 6' table. It was all vacuum tube and I designed the whole thing, and we had these transducers, which were made out of pure copper plates, and we put a mylar, like a very thin insulating plastic, over the plates which had 3000 volts across it that was amplitude-modulated, like a radio transmitter, at about 40 kHz. You would put these plates on your head and you could hear music and sound and other things going through it. I demonstrated it—I was a general class ham radio operator since I was eight years old—and so I went to the is Huston amateur radio club with it and demonstrated it to people—and the person with the Neurophone on could hear music but the other people couldn't hear it. It was a big audience—maybe 500 people—and some of the people way in the back of the room heard the music! We determined that it was some kind of electronic telepathy, and a guy there who was a ham radio operator and a reporter for the Houston Post asked me if he could bring his granddaughter, who suffered an attack of spinal meningitis when she was six months old and was completely deaf—no hearing aid or anything would work on her. And we tried the Neurophone on her, and she started bouncing up and down to the music in time with the rhythm, so he pretty much established that she was hearing with it. He put a story out, and the next day it was on the front pages of 300 major newspapers across the United States—that I had invented this this device that might—might—help deaf people to hear.

Then I wrote my own patent when I was 13. My father worked at Shell Laboratories in Houston and one of the patent lawyers there gave me all the information I needed, and I wrote my own patent and sent it in to the patent office. They refused to give me a patent because they said there was no 'prior art,' which meant that no one had ever invented anything like it before. And I thought well, gee—isn't that what a patent is about?, you know, but no—they said that virtually every invention in the world is an improvement on something that is already known. And so I thought the patent office from the age of When I was 19 I flew to Washington DC with my patent attorney; I had more money than my father because I was a consultant for the government and so they took us into the patent office with my Neurophone. They had an employee there who had been nerve deaf, and who for 15 years hadn't heard anything—no hearing aid would work on him—and they said if you can make him hear we will reopen your patent file, which was closed—it had never been done before in history—and they said we will give you your patent.

So they brought him in and we put the Neurophone on him and had a 78 RPM record player with a record of Maria Callas the opera singer singin, and his favorite singer when he had hearing. And we put it on his head, and then he heard for the first time in 15 years and he broke out in tears, sobbing, and pretty soon all the people in the office –every one of them that was in the room—was sobbing and crying because he could hear for the first time in all those years. It was quite an emotional incident I still get emotional over it. And the U.S. patent office gave me my patent, and later, gave me a special honor for that. And I got my patent on the Neurophone.

The current Neurophones are as powerful as that one

was—we couldn't put it on the market because you can't go putting 3000 volts across people's heads, mainly because if the installation on the electrodes if it had a tear in the insulation or a pinprick hole, it would give them an RF burn on the skull, and so I had to forgo the original design and come up with the digital design. The present Neurophone works really well, but one of the things we discovered is that carrier frequency—there's something called the ultrasonic effect—and it turns out that that when we hear even with our ears, even ultrasonic frequencies way beyond the range of human hearing, that blood flow to the brain is increased, and causes your left and right hemispheres to become more coherent, and also increases transmission of information across the corpus callosum, which is the divider between the left and right hemispheres of the brain. And it turns out that the ultrasonics carrier itself, even without modulation, helps increase blood flow to the brain, and also using acupuncture devices we determined that it that increases balance of the acupuncture meridians and all kinds of things. I put out numerous versions of the Neurophone over the years. At first I was blocked because the Neurophone was subsequently put under secrecy by the NSA and I couldn't sell it, just like the muscle detector I mentioned earlier.

One listener, David. really likes the Megahydrate to structure water. He says, "I think the products are terrific I've been using Megahydrate and Crystal Energy, and found dramatic and excellent hydration, the taste is excellent. Also, it absolutely stimulates and enhances absorption of co-supplements when taken together with them. I see some obvious changes to the skin; we're just overall feeling My wife is has had a liver transplant, which has incurred a total joint replacement along the way, and these products have created a noticeable upswing in several ways. We're very impressed, and thank you. A question—is it okay to mix Megahydrate and Crystal Energy together? And Megahydrate and carbonated water?

PF: You can, you can.

PT: Or Megahydrate with colloidal silver or iodine?

PF: Absolutely.

PT: And finally, any other recommendations to further structure water beyond Mega hydrate and Crystal Energy

PF: The infrared sauna sonic talked about earlier—Dr. Pollock has discovered the infrared wavelengths that help structure and increased capillary flow in the body and I highly recommend that. I wish I could carry one with me. I learned a long time ago when I was very young from my Beverly Hills lawyer, who said first class is less expensive –you want to get a first-class infrared sauna, you don't want to go with something that doesn't have the wavelengths that Dr. Pollock recommends.

PT: Here's a question on ormus homeopathics. . .do you have any theories on that?

PF: David Wolfe is a really good friend of mine—"Avocado" David Wolfe is such an awesome being--he reminds me so much of myself when I was his age—and I've known him for many many years. . . One of the things he did his is—if you add Crystal Energy to water flooded and put it in an ice tray in the icebox, in most cases the water forms stalagmites coming up out of the ice tray, like the water was levitating when it was frozen. He said that's a sign of ormus, because that's one of the ways he tests for ormus—to to put the ormus in water and then freeze it and see what happens with the ice. We even had a video where, when you add Megahydrate and/or Crystal Energy to water you can see the water molecules levitating because ormus possesses levity and, actually, antigravity. David has said the Crystal Energy has the most orumus of anything he has ever tested—so you get you get all that in one-- Crystal Energy is a source of ormus.

PT: The second part of the question is—do you think it's ever going to be possible to reverse hybrid and GMO plants' DNA back to heirloom.

PF: There is actually a way to do that. There was a study where what they did is they took seeds and wet them, and then they put a high voltage across them, with a negative charge on the bottom to represent the earth and a positive plate over the top of the seeds to produce a pretty intense DC, high-voltage field—and what they discovered was that ordinary seeds go back to heirloom condition simply by doing that. The scientist that discovered this also did it with fish eggs; what they did is they took some salmon eggs and fertilized them under high-voltage field the same way until the little fish started the hatch, and the salmon were like salmon that they found in prehistoric fossils, as if they had found skeletons of salmon in What happened is that it turned them back in heirloom fish, so to speak. They published this information, and then what happened is that the company closed the lab and fired the scientists when they discovered and published their findings. Then the scientists set up their own lab on the side and continued to research and then every single one of them except one of the scientists died in an horrific accidents and such things within a year—five scientists all died. The idea behind all this is that these guys were murdered because as they had discovered a way to return seeds into heirloom forms.

PT: A listener asks if there's a way to increase their IQ other than the Neurophone.

PF: I helped develop a device called the neural efficiency analyzer; it's a device that tests IQ electronically because it actually tests an establishes the efficiency of the brain, because ordinary IQ test are most definitely language-oriented--which insults some people who grew up, let's say, in the deep South. There are some very, very primitive areas where people join the military in order to get an education and all that, and so they established this sound neural efficiency analyzer to test IQ and they found out that it was extremely accurate. I helped develop that machine, and one of the things that they did is they tested people and then we'd have them wear the Neurophone for half an hour and then test them again, and it improved their IQ significantly. That's because idt causes the left and right hemispheres to become more phase coherent the higher their IQ the more you're using your brain in a more efficient, effective way.

I've used the Neurophone since I was 13, continuously, and when I was in high school and they tested my IQ they said it was off the charts-- they could not measure my IQ—this was with the written test. They said that my IQ was over 200—I think they called it the Greenlee test or something like that, and the and they said that I showed up with an IQ of 200 and that that was the maximum that they could measure using that particular test. And I have to say that I think it was Neurophone that did that for me.

PT: Here's an email from Jesse: "I bought the $800 Neurophone, and the first night I use it, it was wild—huge, beautiful dreams, past lives. I recommend it highly. Now it's not working as well as it did when I first bought it.

PT: You know the man Germany who manufactures the NF3—his name is Hans Strobel –ever since he got his first Neurophone he has been wearing it for several years 24 hours a day, seven days a week except for when he takes a shower. He wears it when he sleeps, and all he does is change the battery every nine hours or so. He said that it has had the most amazing effect on him ever, and that his dreams are incredible. I would say that this person needs to use the Neurophone at least an hour a day for them to get the best results

PT: On which setting?

PF On the NF3 you just turn it on and can have it on—you don't have to listen to music. I would wet the transducers or use KY jelly—you put a little jelly on the transducers, place them on your forehead, loop the wires behind your ears and listen to the Neurophone especially before you go to sleep. Some people like to wind down for the evening, so they can go to sleep more easily add and add but just put the Neurophone on with the carrier only and listen to it for him for about a about an hour. I often go to sleep with the Neurophone on; I put it on and I fall asleep, and in the middle of the night I'll wake up I'll wake up and turn it off. The new Neurophone actually has a sleep setting you can put it on and it will put you to sleep.

PART 3

ON ARTHRITIS

PT: How would Dr. Flanagan recommend somebody

who is in terrible pain deal reversing rheumatoid arthritis?

PF: Oh, that's sad and—I'm sorry to hear that. I can't tell you what to do—that's called prescribing and you can't prescribe anything over the airways—but if I had rheumatoid arthritis the first thing I would do is try to drink pure distilled water, and I would add things like Crystal Energy to it—but there is an incorrect thought that distilled water takes vital minerals out of the body—it does not. The body will only release minerals it doesn't need or want anymore, except under stress, in which it releases some minerals that are vital to the body. But I would drink distilled water; and then I'd go on as pure a diet as possible, and of course, you take all these wonderful supplements.

ON SCALAR ENERGIES

PT: Another email—they want to know what Dr. Patrick Flanagan thinks about scalar energy and scalar devices.

PF: Well, actually, my book *Pyramid Power*, is about some scalar devices that I made. The pyramid is actually a scalar resonator and if the pyramid structure is made according to the Golden Ratio it actually is a scalar resonator; it increases also resonates to scalar wavelengths that in the Golden Ratio, because all living systems of the human body and the hydrogen bond are all based on the Fibonacci Ratio. And so, happily, I'm very much into scalar—or what are also called longitudinal waves; some people called scalar waves, but more accurately they're termed longitudinal. All of Nicola Tesla's work involved using scalar or longitudinal waves. When I was 30 I invented a scalar communicator and I could actually transmit audio modulated longitudinal waves through a mountain and successfully—so you could transmit through the earth with it without any decrease in intensity—and of course that would be great for submarines and things like that. My guess—because I don't know for sure and so I'm not disclosing anything that's been revealed to me--but my guess is that a lot of the submarine communication devices being used in the world are a longitudinal wave devices or scalar weight devices.

PT: So if you surround yourself something that has scalar energies, it's beneficial?

PF: Oh, absolutely.

ON MEGAHYDRATE AND HYDROGEN

PT: We have a question about a burping reaction to Megahydrate. But you've said before that this response is natural.

PF: Oh, definitely. Some negative people who don't know what they're talking about said that Megahydrate had carbonate—or carbon dioxide—in it, but you're actually burping hydrogen, negative ionized hydrogen. I proved it—there's a video online at buzzbroz showing how I put Megahydrate in a bottle, shook it up and squeezed all the air out of it and waited a while until some of the hydrogen that was released from our product filled the bottle—and when we popped the top of the bottle and put a flame over the top of it, it shot a flame all the way to the ceiling, with the hydrogen burning with some of the oxygen that was already in the bottle. That was my proof that this was hydrogen this is not carbonate.

ON MEGAHYDRATE & MUSCLE PAIN

PT: Dr. Flanagan said he took a Megahydrate for muscle pain; how much did he take and did it take very long to work? He's been having some issues with messed up hip and leg muscles.

PF: That's a little different—you know, athletes, when they exercise really hard, generate.lactic acid, causing muscle pain because they've been exercising. We showed that when you take out Megahydrate before you exercise, it reduces the lactic acid reduces it buy as much is two thirds, and we actually have published an article on that and so we highly recommend it for that; but it if you're having pain because of a displaced disk or an injury—like I've been in motorcycle accidents and all kinds of things and I end up having a lot of pain it in my back and body—and when I was in in a lot of pain the only thing that really helped it is some soma that I got from my doctor—that's carisoprodol. I would take one of those, and naturally I would take my own products but I found out that that it worked just as well as the heavier duty painkillers, and I found that it that just relaxed me enough to take the edge off the pain. Me. But I highly recommend you go to a doctor who is an expert on pain, because some doctors are afraid to handle pain that way because they're afraid you're going to become addicted to pills and so forth. And that's possible, but for the most part people who actually take painkillers just for the purpose of taking the edge off of it is less stressful on your body than avoiding the painkillers. And so that I highly recommend a good pain doctor for some things like that—I'm sorry that I don't have a better answer for you, other than an infrared sauna and other things like that that might help.

ON FREQUENCY SEED TREATMENT

Rexresearch.com would have the articles on the seed treatment

PF: Definitely, you can find it; Rex Research is a wonderful source of. I've known them for 30 or 40 years and I highly recommend them. The guy is an amazing researcher—he goes through all the patents in the office He;s got a lot of a lot of information of me and my life in there—they're off the charts.

PF: It's one of the best sources of information—some stuff in it comes with a charge, but it's very reasonable and definitely worth every bit of it.

ON ACID REFLUX

PT: A listener wants to know if you have any suggestions about dealing with acid reflux. Have you ever had to deal with that over the years?

PF: I have, because I'm short and because sometimes, as you're growing older you shrink a little bit and in your esophagus can move down into your stomach so that some of the acid in your stomach refluxes into your esophagus; one of the things that the that a doctor friend of mine recommended was to drink a whole bunch of water and then bounce up and down in place or on a rebound or trampoline. What it does is it hold your stomach down so that your esophagus is no longer extending into your stomach. That's one thing that actually works. A lot of doctors recommend anti-acid pills, and sometimes it's the only thing you can do, but I don't recommend it because hydrochloric acid is very important for us.

PT: Isn't that a classic hiatal hernia, where you could use the water and get on the rebounder and pull it down?

PF: Exactly, and it does work—the rebounder with water works.

PT: How much water do you have to drink?

PF: I would say—try drinking a liter of water a quart of water.

PT: Have you come across any secrets over the years about the stomach, digestion and the colon?

PF: Well, it depends on how old you are. As we get older we lose some of the enzymes –if you eat foods that digest themselves that's is pretty nice. Raw or lightly steamed steamed foods, especially, often come with their own digestive enzymes. But as we get older sometimes it's good to get a good digestive aid or supplement, like probiotics. That's why Megahydrate is so good, because when we're younger we make our make our own from the food we eat, but as we get older we lose the enzymes. And also with all the attacks on the energy systems of the body in our highly stressful world, Megahydrate and Crystal Energy certainly help a lot with that also.

PT: I can remember seeing a really critical video in which there was a fellow using Megahydrate and all this fancy electronic equipment; he was testing the qualities of water using your Megahydrate, just using a quarter of a capsule!

PF: Yes, it's incredible. By the way, I found my file— it's call "The Cibagigy Effect." It's a Swiss company Cibagigy is one of the largest pharmaceutical companies in the world. They got a European patent on the use of electrostatic fields to treat mushroom seeds, fish and all kinds of things. And it was Heinz Schurch who watched over the experiments until 1992. And I've done some of these experiments, I've created some of these original—you could say--heirloom seeds from ordinary seeds. I haven't tried it with genetic seeds—and if I did I wouldn't say it!

PF: These guys wrote a book—it's in German—in which they show high resolution of the fish, ferns and seeds; and you'll find, if you do the research, these guys all died mysteriously—no one's accusing the pharmaceutical companies of doing that, but it's too bad all these guys doing the research died.

ON RADIATION PROTECTION

PT: What do you think happens when we get exposed to wi-fi, cellphones, cellphone towers and such things?

PF: There are two possibilities: one is that the electromagnetic field strength is so high that it causes your body to 'cook,' but the biggest thing is that the signals from wi-fi and cellphones are pulsing at low frequencies—we're talking about packets of digital data. Pulsing frequency is usually in the range of the brain waves and the nervous system, and what happens is that the body keeps trying to log onto the signals because it thinks it's trying to penetrate into the body. The body thinks that the signal is a biological signal sent out by its own system, and it keeps trying to lock onto it and it's just getting nonsense, and so basically it can screw up some of your biological processes. Andrea Puharich, who was a friend—and in some ways, an enemy—of mine, because he was a psychiatrist who worked for the---discovered that red iron oxide—if you live in Sedona, Arizona, you find makes up much of the surrounding environment, and it makes it a very good place to live.

Recording tapes—like VCR tapes—had a coating of iron oxide. Using an oscillator with a microscope, Puharich discovered that these crystals naturally resonate at what's called Schumann Resonance, which is 7.83 Herz, and it turns out that Schumann Resonance, like everything on earth, evolved for millions of years without radio transmitters, wi-fi or cell phones, and that the body is constantly looking for this 7.83 Herz signal in order to rebalance itself; and Puharich discovered that these iron oxide crystals— and you discover them, in all things, in red Jeweler's Rouge—that these crystals naturally vibrate at 7.83 Herz. So what I did was to take a rapidly drying nail polish some fine Jeweler's Rouge and put it in the nail polish and stirred it up until it was red and then put it back in the bottle and then painted my computer and cell phones with some of this paint—and so now the signals coming from the wi-fi and the cellphone are causing the Jeweler's Rouge to put out a coherent Schumann Resonance signal—and what happens is that the body latches on to the coherent Schumann Resonance signals and says, 'Ah, I can relax and ignore all those other digital signals.' And I've had friends with smart meters tell me they'd take some Jeweler's Rouge and put it into some paint and painted the inside of the wall opposite the place where the smart meter was mounted, and in the case of this one particular guy, whose children and wife were getting sick from the smart meter, walk into the house and say, "What did you do—remove the smart meter?'— and he said "No, I painted the wall," and showed her. His wife was no longer getting migraine headaches, no longer sick, and his children got better. And now we've had a few thousand people do this; it doesn't take a lot—a teaspoon of really fine Jeweler's Rouge polish has literally billions and billions of these crystals in it, and if you painted some on the back of your phone or computer or smart meter it starts to transform the resonant signals and I've had so many people tell me they've had relief from this that I can't but recommend it.

Don't get the Jeweler's Rouge sticks—it must be the red powder. You can get them from Jewelry supply houses or online, but make sure it's the red Jeweler's Rouge powder.

PT: How much do you think you'd have to put into a gallon of paint to make it effective?

PF: Well, this one fellow went all the way and he put— like—a cup of it in there, but I don't think you have to go that far; if you put 2 or 3 teaspoons or tablespoons into a gallon of paint, I think that would be enough. I think that that's plenty.

PT: Is Schumann similar to scalar?

PF: Schumann Resonance—because the earth is a capacitance field—it turns out that the capacitance field between the ionosphere and the earth is a capacitance field, and that Schumann Resonance is the earth's resonant frequency of that capacitor, and what happens is that the earth's field is so weak—because we have so many millions of microwave and other signals from the ionosphere, is that the body is losing track of the resonant frequency. The earth is a scalar field, it is a resonant 7.83 Herz, longitudinal wave—or what some people might call a scalar—field.

Listener: A while ago Patrick Timpone interviewed Tyler LeBaron from the Molecular Hydrogen Foundation, and he was talking about promoting the ionizers that create hydrogen-rich water, sharing that it's important to measure how much dissolved hydrogen is in the water in parts per million. Is there any way we can measure this?

PF: Well, using an Oxidation Reduction Potential meter—or what we call an ORP meter—and there are really good ORP meters that don't use wet bulbs—but, basically, if the water has negative ionized hydrogen it will have a negative ORP—oxidation reduction potential. Pure oxygen has a potential of about 1.24 volts positive, and if you a capsule of Megahydrate into a glass of water you'll usually get a reduction of about 800 millivolts. It will go down to about 700 minus in oxidation reduction potential, and if you're testing these water ionizers, what they call the alkaline water should have a 300 or 400 oxidation reduction potential in a good ionizer. I can say that I highly recommend those ionizers, but if you can't afford one you can certainly buy Megahydrate—it does everything the water ionizers will do.

PT: But couldn't there be some downside to drinking that much alkaline water—doesn't it alkalize it as well as adding hydrogen to it?

PF: Well, no—the water ionizers have an acid side and an alkaline side to them; they recommend the acid water for killing bacteria and such things and they recommend the alkaline water for drinking. The water is not that alkaline; when you get down to it, 5 gallons of ionized, alkaline water doesn't have as much hydrogen as 1 capsule of Megahydrate. A lot of people own the ionizers—I don't own one—who not only take alkaline water but also take Megahydrate just to make sure they're getting enough.

PT: Does Dr. Flanagan have any ways of detoxifying fluoride from the water and the body?

PF: Well, Megahydrate, if added to the water, will neutralize fluoride and chlorine in the water. But I highly recommend a filter that removes fluoride from the water, and I highly recommend drinking distilled water and not getting any fluoride in your body—I don't care if it's from the dentist, or from toothpaste or from the water you drink. I highly recommend you buy a good reverse osmosis device that removes everything, or a water distiller that removes the fluoride and the chlorine. I have personally consumed, when I can, pure reverse osmosis water or distilled water for over the last 50 years.

ON OZONE & HYPERBARIC OXYGEN

Caller: What does Dr. Flanagan think about ozone, either ozonated water or through rectal insufflation.

PF: Well I also recommend ozone, but I also recommend that you take Megahydrate before you do the ozone therapy, because ozone does crate free radicals that the body has to deal with, as does hyperbaric oxygenation. I highly recommend ozone enemas or ozone water enemas, ozone as a water treatment. I'm all for ozone therapy, it's an excellent therapy.

PT: Do you think hyperbaric sessions are worth the cost?

PF: I do, especially if you take Megahydrate before you go into the chamber.

PT: Can Dr. Flanagan please discuss fourth phase water, and how it works in the cells and in the body.

PF: When you add Crystal Energy to water, it actually creates fourth phase water around all the little crystal energy colloids, Dr. Pollack is familiar with our product but he cannot recommend products—he has to maintain his neutrality as a university professor— but he's tested our product. It helps to produce fourth phase water, which is highly structured water; fourth phase water has a negative redox potential. A far infrared sauna helps to make it in the body; adding Crystal Energy to water helps to make it in your body when the water is taken. I highly admire Dr. Pollack and his work.

THE MIRACLE OF MEGAHYDRATE

Hydrogen is the key to everything. It is the first element in the chart of elements and some could say the foundation for the entire universe. It is the first atom, giving birth to all other atoms. We like to think of it as the mother of form.

Much could be said about hydrogen, but really what Megahydrate does is have the safest, healthiest, most powerful form of stabilizing free electrons, also known as, antioxidants. Free radicals are what wreak havoc in our bodies and they do that by stripping electrons from everything they come in contact with.

This is one of the major factors in aging and ill health, the damage caused from free radicals. The remedy? Electrons. Free electrons that can be given from one molecule to another without turning the previous into a free radical itself. Most "anti-oxidants", such as ascorbic acid (vitamin C), do exactly that though.

The form that is left behind after they neutralize a free radical actually becomes a free radical itself, only now is less harmful and easier to remove from the body than what it just neutralized.

Why is Megahydrate the most powerful antioxidant known to man?

Because its one of the only things that we know of that doesn't turn into a free radical after neutralizing other free radicals. The bi-product is hydrogen, which then binds with oxygen to create water. Its greatest secret however, is that it converts every other antioxidant, turned free radical itself, back into an antioxidant that it comes in contact with. This is called "replenishing the anti-oxidant cascade".

Did you catch that? It replenishes every other anti-oxidant in the entire anti-oxidant cascade back into an antioxidant!

That is why it is the most powerful anti-oxidant known to mankind!

MegaHydrate is the key that unlocks the potential of water as the medium for nutrient replenishment and waste removal at the cellular level. In a state of dehydration, body cells cannot assimilate nutrients and remove waste and relieve pain from conditions like arthritis or fibromyalgia.

Dehydration also occurs as a side effect of caffeine. Caffeine effects include anxiety, dizziness, headaches, sleep disorders, and many common ailments. MegaHydrate also helps fight the negative effects of alcohol, stress, and free radicals as part of aging. In addition to hydration, MegaHydrate is the most powerful known antioxidant food.

Since it is an "pure" antioxidant that does not turn into a free radical itself, taken daily, MegaHydrate delivers far more Hydrogen ions than eating pounds of raw fruits and vegetables or drinking gallons of "healing waters," also known as "glacial milk." Humans need Hydrogen to survive. It is the key to long life and anti-aging.

However, due to mass food production, mineral deficient soil, pesticides, chemical fertilizers, over-processing of foods, chemical preservatives, and drinking over-chlorinated and over-fluoridated water, people do not get enough Hydrogen ions daily. Body cells become damaged, hydration levels decrease and cells age.

In summary, MegaHydrate challenges the symptoms of dehydration and minimizes the process of aging. Many customers report immediate pain relief and increases in energy. MegaHydrate is a dietary supplement that is considered a food grade supplement rich in antioxidants by the FDA.

Antioxidant foods like MegaHydrate help defy the aging process. It is safe, having been tested and shown to have no known side effects.

JOSEPH MARCELLO

Patrick Flanagan - Scientific biography

According to his biography, Patrick Flanagan, who was born on Oct. 11, 1944 (22 months after Nikola Tesla died), "invented the Neurophone in 1958. It is an electronic nervous system excitation device that transmits sound through the skin directly to the brain, for which he received U.S. Patent no.3,393,279 in 1968.

"The invention earned him a profile in Life magazine, which called him a "unique, mature and inquisitive scientist". Flanagan has continued to develop the Neurophone and it is currently being sold as an aid to speed learning.

"Flanagan at age eleven developed and sold a guided missile detector to the U.S. Military, aged seventeen gained his air pilot's license and was employed by a Think Tank at The Pentagon, and later as a consultant to the NSA, CIA, NASA, Tufts University, the Office of Naval Research, and the Aberdeen Proving Grounds for the Department of Unconvential Weapons and Warfare.

"Since 1981 Flanagan has invented a series of useful devices and products based on water and specific mineral structures, in the area of health. Several of these have been very successful in the marketplace. His identification of the special properties of the negative hydride ion while once ridiculed got serious attention when the Nobelist Chandrasekhar proposed it as a major component in far space. Several scientific papers by Flanagan, about Silica Hydride have been published in peer reviewed journals such as the 'International Journal of Hydrogen Energy', and 'Free Radical Biology and Medicine'.

"Flanagan actively continues his activities as scientist and inventor and philanthropist, promoting the really new science and new approaches to human healing, especially those based on the great traditions of India and Egypt."

THE AUTHOR

Joseph Marcello is an award-winning composer who has explored paths to awakening since early adolescence, studying, in addition to Douglas Harding, with such mentors as Karlfried Graf von Durckheim in the Black Forest, author of *Hara, the Vital Centre of Man*, Krishnamurti's protégé, Vimala Thakar, whose awakening is documented in her *On an Eternal Voyage*, Sachindra Majumdar in New York, author of *Yoga, Principles & Practices*, and Paramhansa Yogananda's disciple, Roy Eugene Davis, author of *This is Reality*.

He has authored and edited some 8 books on well-being, subtle energies and awakening, including *Life More Abundant; the Science of Zhineng Qigong, Living Vision—the Secret Teachings of Neville Goddard, The Healing Power of Pyramids, Elixir of the Ageless* and *The Hindu Secrets of Virility & Rejuvenation*. He lives on a pine clad hill in Western Massachusetts just below the New Hampshire and Vermont borders, and adores the shoulder-to-shoulder presence of the twenty-odd cockatiels and parakeets he has bred and hand-fed through 5 generations of lineage.

He may be contacted at: JosephMarcello@verizon.net.

JOSEPH MARCELLO

FLANAGAN SPEAKS!

JOSEPH MARCELLO